Volleyball Today

Second Edition

Marv Dunphy
Pepperdine University

Rod Wilde
United States Men's National Team

Series Editor
Bob O'Connor, Ed. D.

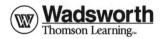 **Wadsworth**
Thomson Learning™

Australia • Canada • Denmark • Japan • Mexico • New Zealand • Philippines
Puerto Rico • Singapore • South Africa • Spain • United Kingdom • United States

Publisher: Peter Marshall
Editorial Assistant: Keynia Johnson
Project Editor: Matt Stevens
Print Buyer: Barbara Britton
Permissions Editor: Robert M. Kauser
Production: Fritz/Brett Associates Inc.
Interior and Cover Designer: Harry Voigt Graphic

Copyeditor: Elaine Brett
Illustrator: Carole Lawson
Cover Image: Jeff Stork and Craig Buck; reprinted with
permission from the United States Volleyball Association
Compositor: Pat Rogondino
Printer/Binder: Webcom Ltd.

Printed in Canada

1 2 3 4 5 6 03 02 01 00 99

Library of Congress
Cataloging-in-Publication Data
Dunphy, Marv.
    Volleyball today / Marv Dunphy, Rod Wilde. -- 2nd ed.
    p. cm. -- (Wadsworth's physical education series)
    Includes index.
    ISBN 0-534-35836-5 (pbk.)
    1. Volleyball--United States. I. Wilde, Rod. II. Title. III.
Series.
    GV1015.55.D86 2000
    796.325'0973--dc21
                                    99-33874

Wadsworth/Thomson Learning
10 Davis Drive
Belmont, CA 94002-3098
USA
www.wadsworth.com

International Headquarters
Thomson Learning
290 Harbor Drive, 2nd Floor
Stamford, CT 06902-7477
USA

UK/Europe/Middle East
Thomson Learning
Berkshire House
168-173 High Holborn
London WC1V 7AA
United Kingdom

Asia
Thomson Learning
60 Albert Street #15-01
Albert Complex
Singapore 189969

Canada
Nelson/Thomson Learning
1120 Birchmount Road
Scarborough, Ontario M1K 5G4
Canada

Contents

Wadsworth's Physical Education Series

Aerobics Today, by Carole Casten and Peg Jordan
Aqua Aerobics Today, by Carol Casten
Badminton Today, by Tariq Wadood and Karlyne Tan
Golf Today, 2nd edition, by J. C. Snead and John L. Johnson
Jazz Dance Today, by Lorraine Person Kriegel and Kim Chandler-Vaccaro
Racquetball Today, by Lynn Adams and Erwin Goldbloom
Swimming and Aquatics Today, by Ron Ballatore, William Miller, and Bob O'Connor
Strength Training Today, 2nd edition, by Bob O'Connor, Jerry Simmons, and J. Patrick O'Shea
Tennis Today, 2nd edition, by Glenn Bassett, William Otta, and Christine Shelton
Volleyball Today, 2nd edition, by Marv Dunphy and Rod Wilde

The Series Editor for Wadsworth's Physical Education Series

Dr. Bob O'Connor received his B.S. and M.S. degrees in physical education from UCLA and his doctorate from U.S.C. His 40-year teaching experience includes instruction in physical education courses for tennis, weight training, volleyball, badminton, swimming, and various team sports, as well as classes in teaching methods. Internationally, Dr. O'Connor has been an advisor to several Olympic programs in weight training and swimming. He was among the first to popularize strength training for all athletic events. Dr. O'Connor has written extensively in the fields of physical education and health.

Preface

It is our fervent hope that this book will present an approach to learning the game of volleyball that will rapidly take the learner from basic beginner play to the intermediate or advanced levels. The more quickly the player gets to a high level of play, the greater his or her enjoyment of the game.

We have attempted to explain the techniques and strategies that we teach in our beginning, intermediate, and advanced classes and in our instructional camps. To some people it may seem that the skills presented here are more than beginning level. Since every student learns at a different pace, there may be too much material for some and not enough for others. For that reason we have presented in each fundamental chapter a checklist for progression of learning.

The fundamentals and team play of volleyball have rapidly evolved, as has the method of teaching. The pedagogy of teaching skills has been found to be much more effective in a game-related situation than in non-game-related drills.

Acknowledgments

The development of this text could not have progressed without the helpful criticism and suggestions from colleagues. We gratefully acknowledge the reviewers of this edition: Sharon King, University of California at Davis; Brock D. Knight, Arizona State University; Colleen Riley, Fullerton College; and Tim Toon, Walla Walla Community College. We would also like to acknowledge our collegues who reviewed the first edition: Patti Barrett, Southwest Texas State University; Ed Bigham, Southern Illinois University Dave Markland, University of North Carolina; Elaine Michaelis, Brigham Young University; Edlin Onsgard, Los Angeles Pierce College; and Tom Peterson, Pennsylvania State University.

Thanks also to players Glenn Sato, Nina Mathies, Rick McLaughlin, and Elaine Roque, who served as models for the text photographs, and to David Hanover, Christine Kranzler, and Gerhard Pagels for their excellent photography.

Grateful thanks to Christine Wells for her input in the nutrition, diet, and mental conditioning chapters. Her extensive work in these areas has been a major contribution to the book.

Marv Dunphy
Rod Wilde

Foreword

Marv Dunphy is an outstanding teacher. This statement has been earned and proven by directing gold medal success at both collegiate and Olympic levels. Success in team sports is always the result of the players being taught the ability to properly and quickly execute the individual fundamentals and channel their abilities into the team concept. Coach Dunphy has shown an ability to do this second to none. Every coach and every player can greatly enhance their ability by carefully studying the techniques explained in this book.

Coach John Wooden
Ten-time NCAA National Champion Coach

1   *The Game of Volleyball*

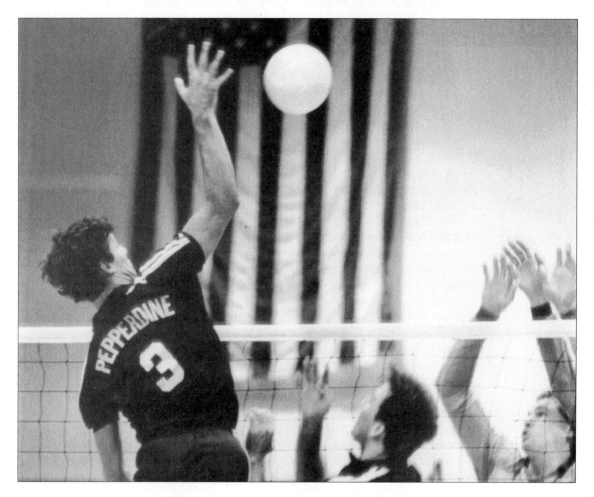

Outline

Volleyball has become a very popular game in America and throughout the world. It is the world's second most popular sport, second only to soccer. It is played from elementary school age through the senior citizen ranks. It is played with as few as two players per team to as many as six in official games, and sometimes even more in pickup games and at picnics.

It is an international game that requires great skill and complex strategy, but it can be adapted to any level of play—and it is always fun.

History

The game was first developed by William G. Morgan who had completed his degree in physical education in 1894 at Springfield College, then known as the School for Christian Workers. While working at a YMCA (Young Men's Christian Association) in Holyoke, Massachusetts, he attempted to get the local businessmen involved in the game of basketball, which had also been developed by a Springfield College man.

Morgan succeeded in getting some men interested in playing basketball for recreation, but some of the older men didn't like the game's roughness. Morgan then thought of just having them hit the basketball back and forth by hand. He also considered having them play tennis, but rejected the idea because the equipment required (balls, racquets, and nets) was too costly. But the concept of a net to divide the players seemed like a good idea, so he put a net between two groups of participants. He decided to put the net at a height of six and a half feet. (It is now near eight feet.) Next he developed a few rules and a new game was developed.

Games usually don't evolve in vacuums. The game of *minton* was probably familiar to Morgan—it might be considered a first cousin to volleyball. Minton was introduced into the United States in 1895. The game was played by two teams of four players who played on a 40 x 80 foot court and hit the ball over the net with a bat. The net was six to six and a half feet high. The server would hit the ball over the net and a returner would have to immediately hit it back over. If the server's team failed to get the ball over, it was a fault and the server lost the serve. If the returners failed to return the ball, the serving team got a point. When all players on the serving team had lost their serves, the side would be out and the other team would get the serve. When both sides were out it was called the completion of an inning. Four innings constituted a game[1].

Morgan's group first tried hitting a basketball, which was too heavy, then a basketball bladder, which was too light and slow. Because the basketball was

---

[1]"Minton," *YMCA Athletic League Handbook*, New York: American Sports Publishing Co., 1897, p. 168.

"too heavy and made our wrists sore, . . . we had Spaulding Company make us a ball made of soft calfskin which didn't last long[2]."

While Morgan said that he had no knowledge of any similar games, there were actually a few European sports that were somewhat like his. During the Middle Ages, groups of Italians played a game that had some similarities to volleyball. A modification of that game, introduced into Germany in 1893, was called *faust ball*.

Morgan first called his game *mintonette*. The first exhibition of the game was at Springfield College on July 7, 1896. Among the participants at the first game were J. Curran and John Lynch, respectively the mayor and fire chief of Holyoke.

In 1896 Morgan was invited to give a demonstration of the game to a conference at Springfield College. He gave the presider a copy of the rules of the game—written in long hand[3].

While watching the game at Springfield College, faculty member Alfred Halstead christened the game "volleyball." It seemed like a logical name because the ball was volleyed over the net.

The rules changed often. In the original game, as in today's game, any number of players could play, the ball had to be volleyed, not caught, and the players could not touch the net. Other rules were different. The court size was not standardized, and players did not rotate.

In 1896, W. E. Day introduced the new sport at Dayton, Ohio. He developed some new rules. Among the rule changes were that the net was raised to seven and one-half feet, eliminating the possibility of dribbling the ball (multiple hits by one player), and that the game was standardized at 21 points.

The more modern version of the rules started in 1912. The court and the ball were standardized, and the rule requiring the players to rotate before a serve was instituted. In 1916, the YMCA and the NCAA (National Collegiate Athletic Association) published the rules of the game and made additional changes. They set the height of the net at eight feet, set the game score at 15, and made the winner of the match the team that won two out of three games.

In the early 1920s, A. Provost Idell and his teammates added a few more rules. They standardized the court at 30 x 60 feet, established the rule limiting the number of hits per side to three, and required that the ball be played only from above the waist.

Popularity

Volleyball began to become popular. The game was introduced to the Phillipines in 1910, to Japan in 1913, to Poland in 1915, to Uruguay in 1916, to

---

[2] George O. Draper, "William C. Morgan—Inventor of Volleyball," *Official Volleyball Rules*, New York: American Sports Publishing Co., 1970, p. 41.

[3] Ibid.

Brazil and Latvia in 1919, and to Syria in 1922. After World War I, it was introduced throughout Europe.

While the YMCA kept volleyball as an indoor game, the Playground of America (now the National Recreation Association) started to teach it as an outdoor game after their convention in 1907.

In the early 1920s, the University of Illinois began to teach volleyball as a physical education activity. The university also began an intramural program featuring volleyball competition.

The first college team was started in Oregon in 1928. The University of Washington followed with a team in 1934. These teams played in recreational leagues. The first university volleyball league began in 1941 with 12 teams, among them teams from Columbia, Temple, and the University of Pennsylvania.

By the late 1940s many colleges fielded club teams, and by 1952 the NCAA was willing to sponsor national championships if eight schools were ready to field varsity teams. While many colleges fielded club teams, only six were ready with varsity teams at that time.

The United States Volleyball Association (USVBA) was formed in 1928, and by 1937 it controlled the game in the United States. In 1947, the International Volleyball Federation was formed to regulate the game throughout the world. Fifteen nations sent representatives. (Today there are more than 150 members.) By 1953 the first World Championships were held, in 1955 volleyball was played in the first Pan American Games, and in 1964 it became an Olympic sport.

The popularity of the game today is evidenced by the rapid increase in players. A recent poll showed that 800 million people in the world now play volleyball at least once a week. Of the 50 sports listed in the survey, volleyball was the twelfth most popular sport. Further, the poll showed that in the last 25 years the sport had increased in popularity by 500 percent and that it is growing even more rapidly today, with 46 million Americans now playing the game. The increasing popularity over the years can be credited to the YMCA and physical education programs in high schools and colleges. In fact, more people now participate in volleyball than in tennis, soccer, skiing, racquetball, golf, or baseball.

While the game is most popular among the 25 to 35 age group, it is quickly attracting a following among the young. During the last five years youth volleyball has doubled in popularity and is the fastest-growing sport among young Americans. Interscholastic volleyball is the third most popular sport for girls. And boys teams are rapidly being implemented across the country. In one recent year more than 50 boys' teams were instituted in New York City alone!

As spectator sports, the international game and the beach game continue to attract fans both at the game and on television. As the spectators' knowledge of the game increases, the demand increases for more games. And the demands of television have even influenced rule changes designed to fit the volleyball game into a specific time dimension.

Summary

1. The game of volleyball was invented by William Morgan, a graduate of Springfield College—the same college at which basketball was invented.
2. The game began as a noncontact recreational pastime.
3. The modern rules were fairly well established by the early 1920s.
4. Volleyball is a sport whose popularity is rapidly growing both as a participant sport and as a spectator sport.

2 *Facilities and Equipment*

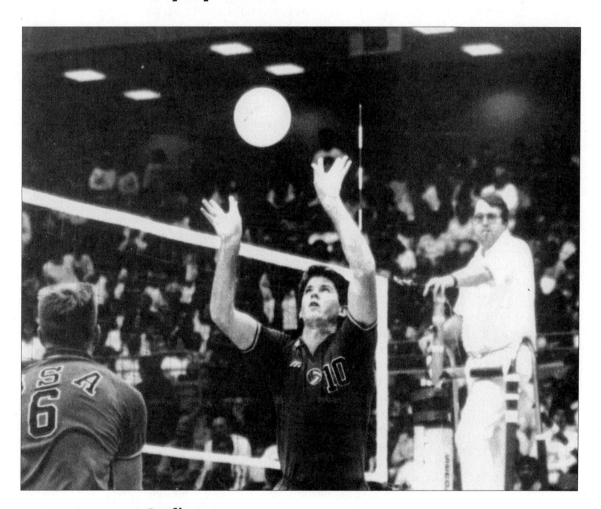

Outline

This chapter describes the physical specifications for volleyball—the dimensions of the court and net, the type of ball to use, and preferred clothing for players.

The Court

The traditional American court is 30 x 60 feet, with a ceiling height of at least 23 feet. With the exception of international matches, most games in the United States are played on this traditional court.

The international court is 59 feet (18 meters) long and 29 and one-half feet wide (nine meters). It is bounded by lines two inches wide. The outside edge of the lines marks the outside perimeter of the court, so the lines are considered inside the court and balls that hit the lines are considered "in." This is different from some games, such as football, where the lines are "out."

There is another line—the center line—that bisects the court into two sections. The net goes over this line. There is also another line on each side of the court running parallel to the net (and center line), three meters from the center line. This is called the "three-meter line," the "back court spiking line," or the "attack line." The three players whose positions were in the back court at the serve cannot contact the ball above net height if the ball is hit over the net. This restrains a team from having its best spiker always playing in the front line.

The serving area is behind the end line and within three meters (ten feet) of the right sideline (as the server faces the net).

The Net

The net is slightly longer than the width of the court; 32 feet is a common length. Most nets are 36 inches from top to bottom, with the cords (made of nylon or other fibers) spaced three to four inches apart so that there is a rather wide mesh (as opposed to a tennis net, which has a narrow mesh). There is a nylon wire cable 1/8- to 3/8-inch in diameter that runs through the top binding of the net. This allows the net to be pulled tightly so that it is nearly straight across.

When set up, the middle of the net will be 8 feet for the traditional American men's game or, for men's international play, 7 feet 11-5/8 inches (2.43 meters) high. For women, the net height is 7 feet 4-1/4 inches in America and 7 feet 4-1/8 inches (2.24 meters) for international play. New rules allow the net to be set at different levels for lower levels of play.

The bottom binding of the net will also be securely anchored. This allows balls that are hit into the net to bounce outward and remain in play.

The Standards

The standards that support the net are mounted in the floor in some gyms. This is the best and safest type of standard. Many gyms have standards that rest on a base on the floor. These require additional anchoring with guy wires set into the floor or the walls.

The Referee's Stand

The referee's stand is generally attached to one of the standards and allows the referee to stand about four feet above floor level. From this vantage point the official can better see the play at the net and can call net touching and illegal movements over or under the net.

The Antennae

In official games a thin pole, usually fiberglass, is extended over the sideline from the top of the net to a level three feet above the net. The antennae are there to assist the officials and players in determining whether or not the ball passed over the net in bounds (inside the antennae). If a team does not hit the ball over the net in bounds, the ball is not in play.

The Ball

The official ball is made of leather and is 25 to 27 inches in circumference. Since 1998, the official rules call for the ball to have alternating white, blue, and yellow panels for good visibility. Because of the cost of leather and the fact that school volleyball is often played outside, manufacturers have developed both synthetic leather balls and rubber balls. Synthetic leather balls cost about half of what leather balls cost, and rubber balls cost only about 25 percent as much as leather balls. Rubber balls also wear better when the game is played on asphalt or concrete. The best-quality balls are softer to the touch because they have more "give" than the harder rubber or synthetic balls. A good ball is a good investment.

Clothing

Shorts and Shirt

A player's shorts and shirt should fit loosely to allow a full range of movement. They should also allow for absorption of perspiration. A blend of 50 percent cotton and 50 percent polyester makes an effective fabric.

Socks

Cotton gym socks should be sufficient. Two pairs of socks help reduce the possibility of getting blisters, because the socks rub against each other and absorb the friction that might otherwise be transferred to your skin.

Checklist for Shoes and Socks

1. Whether you are wearing one or two pairs of socks, pull them up tight so that no wrinkles remain (they might cause blisters).
2. When lacing your shoes, pull the laces tight at the lowest eyelets. Then slowly pull the laces tight at each eyelet upward until the laces have been adjusted at each level. Then tie your laces.
3. Just slipping on your shoes and pulling the laces from the top does not adjust your shoes properly for an action game such as volleyball. Improper lacing can cause blisters.

Shoes

At lower levels of play, nearly any court shoe should be sufficient. Shoes should be pliable, well cushioned, and have good traction. A heel and toe lock will lengthen the life of the shoe. The shoe should also be somewhat rounded to allow for lateral movements. If you are playing indoors, your shoes should have soles that will not mark the floor. At higher levels of play, you may want to buy shoes specifically designed for volleyball.

Sweat Clothes

When you are warming up or playing on cold days, you should wear sweat clothing. Muscles react better and are less susceptible to injury when they are kept warm. Sweats can be worn during a game and should be worn between games or when you are waiting to play. A hooded sweatshirt without a zipper is considered best for volleyball.

Pads

For players who dive for balls, both knee and elbow pads may be worn. They reduce the chance of developing bone bruises or abrasions from contact with the floor. Hip pads are another type of optional equipment that can reduce the chance of injury.

Ankle Braces

Ankle injuries can occur when attackers and blockers jump, often landing on other's feet, so ankle braces, which prevent the foot from being forcibly turned inward, are a wise protective device. They should definitely be used by anyone who has had an ankle sprain, but they are also effective in preventing future sprains. These braces can be purchased in most sporting goods stores. (An ankle brace is made of stiff material or plastic. Elastic compression sleeves do not prevent sprains, and should be used only to reduce swelling after an ankle injury.)

Sweatbands

Some players use sweatbands to keep perspiration from dropping into their eyes. Sweatbands can also be used to keep your hair away from your face.

Other Considerations

Jewelry shouldn't be worn during play; official rules forbid it. A bracelet or wrist watch may break if the ball hits it. Hard objects, such as casts, should also not be worn.

Summary

1. The international court is 18 by 9 meters. The typical American court is 30 x 60 feet. The lines are in bounds.
2. The net height is 7 feet, 11-5/8 inches in the center of the net for men's volleyball and 7 feet 4-1/8 inches for the women's game.
3. Players should wear comfortable clothing (shorts and shirts), perspiration-absorbing socks, and court shoes with good traction and effective shock-absorbing ability.
4. For safety, players may wear knee, elbow, and hip pads to prevent injuries and sweat clothes to prevent pulled muscles.

3

Rules, Regulations, and Terminology

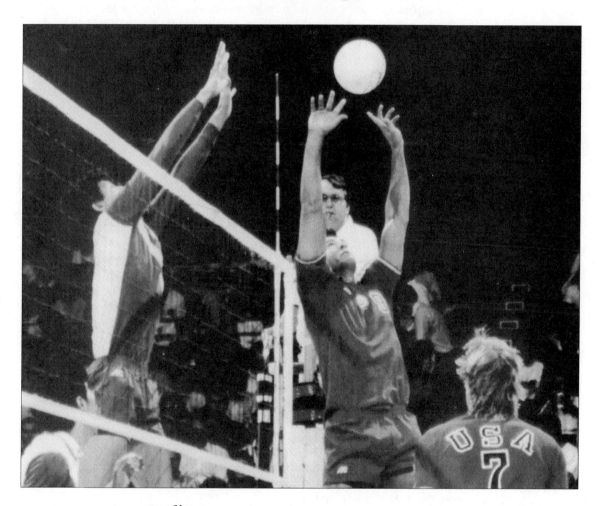

Outline

Rules often change, so players must keep current. For example, it was once allowed to kick the ball; then it was not legal, but now it is legal again. It was once required that players stay in prescribed areas during a serve; now it is required only that they not overlap one another. At one time players were not allowed to cross the plane of the net; now, with certain limitations, they can go over or under as long as they do not touch the net.

The rules vary somewhat from international and college rules to high school, coed, or beach rules. The following rules are for international and college levels of play. However, there are other sanctioning bodies that also make rules. The NAGWS (National Association for Girls' and Women's Sports) formulates the rules for most collegiate women's programs and for some high school girls' competition.

Rules

A *team* is made up of six players. Generally, a squad may have a total of 12 players on the roster; however, some leagues and conferences allow for a variation in this roster rule.

An *official game* is concluded when one team has scored 15 points and has won by two points. In international rules and in men's intercollegiate rules the game is "capped" when a team reaches 17 points, even if it is only one point ahead. Other levels of play have not yet adopted this rule.

The deciding game in a five-game match is a fast-scoring (rally point scoring) game. This means that both teams can score at any time. The serving team scores as it always does, but the receiving team also gains a point when it gets a side out. This obviously speeds up the deciding game.

A *match* is won when one team has won three games out of five or, in a "short match," when one team has won two games out of three.

Flipping the coin for choice of side or serve is done by the captains before the first game and again before the fifth game if a fifth game is needed. The winning captain can choose to serve or to start the game on a preferred side of the court. The position of the sun or a glare from windows might prompt a captain to choose "side" rather than "serve."

Opening serve for the first game is decided by the captain winning the coin toss. For each additional game, the service is alternated. For the final game of a match, such as the fifth game in a best three out of five games, there is another coin toss to determine side or serve.

Points are scored only by the serving team. They are scored when the opponents have committed a foul or the ball lands out of bounds. (In "fast-scoring," either team can score on any serve.)

Side out occurs when the serving team commits a foul or hits the ball out of bounds, thus losing its serve. The opposing team then becomes the serving team.

Positions and zones are named to identify where players are to be during a serve or to determine where a set will be directed or a spike will be hit. The players in the three front zones are called the *right front* (zone 2), *center front* (zone 3), and *left front* (zone 4). The three back row players are the *left back* (zone 5), the *center back* (zone 6), and the server or *right back* (zone 1).

Rotations occur just after a side out as the new server moves from the right front (zone 2) to the right back (zone 1). Players rotate clockwise.

Two *time outs* are allowed to each team per game. Time outs are 30 seconds long.

Substitutions can be made only twice a game (USA rules) or six times per game (international rules). Under these rules the player who was replaced by the substitute must take his or her original position if he or she returns to the game. A starting player can be replaced only one time per game. The substitute cannot return to the game once he or she is replaced by the original player. Most other levels of volleyball allow for 12 substitutions per game.

A *first contact* occurs when a player handles a serve or attack hit. In the first contact, the player may hit the ball with any part of the body.

The allowed *number of contacts* of the ball is limited to three times on each side of the net. A fourth contact would be a foul. So a pass, set, then attack hit would be the three normal contacts that a team would make. The ball can be hit over the net with fewer than three contacts, but not more than three. A block is not counted as one of the three contacts.

Fouls or *violations* result in a side out if committed by the serving team. If they are committed by the receiving team, they result in a point for the serving team.

A violation of any of the following at time of serve results in a side out:

- When the serve is gained, the serving team players rotate clockwise, and the player entering the right back position is the new server.
- The serve must be hit by the right back court player.
- The serve must be hit from an area behind the end line and the server must not be farther back from the end line than nine yards (eight and one-half meters) when serving.
- The server may not step on the back line until after the ball has been contacted.
- The ball must be tossed into the air prior to contacting it with the serving hand.
- The ball can be hit with the hand in any manner.
- The serve cannot hit the net.
- The serve must pass over the net between the antennae.
- Only one service attempt is allowed. If the server drops the ball without hitting it, it is not a foul, and he or she is allowed one more opportunity.
- The serve must land on or between the lines of the receiver's court or be contacted by a player on the receiving team in order to be a legal serve.
- During a serve or service return, a player may not overlap an adjacent player. Thus a back row player cannot be as near the net as the front row player in the zone ahead. And a player cannot overlap the player in the zone to the

side. Once the serve is contacted, the players may move anywhere, but back row players cannot block or spike from ahead of the three meter line.

- A served ball cannot be blocked or spiked by the receiving team. The serving team is awarded a point if this occurs.

A violation of any of the following with the ball in play results in a side out if committed by the serving team or in a point for the serving team if committed by the receiving team:

- Each contact must give the ball immediate impetus. The ball must be clearly hit, not lifted, scooped, or thrown.
- A player may not hit the ball twice in succession (a double hit), unless the first contact was a block, a pass where the fingers do not touch the ball, or a simultaneous hit with another player.
- The ball can be played with any part of the body.
- If opponents hit the ball simultaneously, either can hit it again.
- If teammates hit the ball simultaneously, either can play the next contact.
- The ball may not be hit more than three times in succession by the players of one team, unless the first contact was a block (which does not count as one of the three allowed contacts).
- A team must allow its opponents the opportunity to contact the ball three times on their side of the net. After the ball has been contacted three times, the defenders may reach over the net to block the attacking shot.
- If the ball is partially over the net, it can be contacted by either team.
- The ball must land within the opponents' court or touch any part of the boundary line in order to be called "in bounds."
- Players may not touch the net unless it has been driven into them; however, the ball may touch the net and remain in play (except for a served ball).
- Players may shift positions after the ball has been served, but a player who was in the back row at the time of the service cannot spike or block the ball from inside the three meter line.
- A ball may not be spiked unless part of it has crossed the net. It cannot be touched if it is still on the opponent's side of the net unless the opponent has made the third contact or the ball is clearly going to pass over the net (it can then be blocked).
- Blockers may reach over the net to block a spike after it has been hit. They cannot block a set.
- A player can play under the net if the ball has been hit there by a teammate and has not completely crossed the center line.
- The ball may be played by a player who is out of bounds, but it must cross the net in bounds (completely inside the antennae or the vertical extension of the antennae) in order to be legal.
- No part of the body, other than the foot, may touch the opponent's court. The foot may touch the opponent's court, but some part of the foot must be on or above the center line.

A point must be *replayed* in either of the following instances:

- If two opponents simultaneously hit a ball and the ball is stopped or held the point is replayed.
- If teams make simultaneous fouls the serve is replayed.

 Checklist for Overlap

1. During a serve, before the ball is contacted, the players may not overlap an adjacent player.
   a. The left front player must be positioned so that the left back player is behind and the center front player is to the right.
   b. The center front player must be ahead of the center back player and must not overlap the left or the right front players.
   c. The right front player must be ahead of the right back player and must not overlap the center front player.
   d. The left back player must not be ahead of the left front player and must not overlap the center back player.
   e. The center back player must not line up ahead of the center front player nor overlap either of the other back row players.
   f. The right back player (server) must not be positioned ahead of the right front player nor overlap the center back player.
2. Once the serve is contacted, the players may move to any desired position as long as a back row player does not attempt to block or attack from in front of the three meter line.

Terminology

Ace. An in-bounds legal serve that the opponents cannot return, resulting in a point for the serving team.

Antenna. The vertical rods along the outside edge of the net; they extend 32 inches above the net and indicate out of bounds along the sideline.

Assist. Passing or setting the ball to a teammate, who attacks the ball for a kill.

Attack. The offensive action of hitting the ball; the attempt by one team to terminate the play by hitting the ball to the floor on the opponent's side.

Attack block. Receiving players' aggressive attempts to block a spiked ball before it crosses the net.

Attack line. A line three meters from the net; the attack line separates the front-row players from the back-row players.

Attacker. Also "hitter" and "spiker"; a player who attempts to hit a ball offensively with the purpose of terminating play in his or her team's favor.

Back-row attack. An attack in which a back-row player jumps from behind the nine meter line and attacks the ball.

Back set. A set made when the setter's back is toward the hitter.

Beach dig. An open-handed hit of the ball.

Block. A defensive play by one or more players meant to intercept a spiked ball; the combination of one, two, or three players jumping in front of the opposing spiker and contacting the spiked ball with the hands.

Bump. Descriptive slang for forearm passing.

Bump pass. The use of joined forearms to pass or set a ball in an underhand manner.

Center line. The line directly under the net that divides the court into two equal halves.

Closing the block. The responsibility of the assisting blocker(s) to angle the body relative to the first blocker.

Cross-court shot. An individual attack directed at an angle from one end of the offensive team's side of the net to the opposite sideline of the defensive team's court.

Cut shot. A spike from the hitter's strong side that travels at a sharp angle across the net.

Decoy. An offensive play meant to disguise the spiker who will receive the set.

Deep set. A set to be hit away from the net to confuse the blockers.

Dig. Passing a spiked or rapidly hit ball; slang for the art of retrieving an attacked ball close to the floor.

Dink. Also "tip"; a legal push of the ball around or over blockers.

Double block. Two players working in unison to intercept a ball at the net.

Double hit. Successive hits by the same player (illegal).

Double quick. Two hitters approaching the setter for a quick inside hit.

Doubles. A game with two players on a side.

Down ball. A ball the blockers elect not to attempt to block because it has been set too far from the net or the hitter is not under control.

Five-one. An offensive system that uses five hitters and one setter.

Five set. Set to the right front hitter with a back set.

Flair. Inside-out path of an outside spiker who hid behind a quick hitter.

Floater. A serve with no spin that follows an erratic path.

Forearm pass. A pass in which the player's arms are joined from the elbows to the wrists; the player strikes the ball with the fleshy part of his or her forearms in an underhand motion.

Foul. A violation of the rules.

Four set. A set one foot from the sideline, and on to two feet above the net.

Four-two. An offensive system using four hitters and two setters.

Free ball. A ball that will be returned by a pass rather than a spike; the receiving team should move into serve receive positions.

Held ball. A ball that comes to rest during contact, resulting in a foul.

Hit. To jump and strike the ball with a forceful overhand shot.

Hitter. Also "spiker" or "attacker"; the player who is responsible for hitting the ball.

Inside shoot. A play set; a 33.

Isolation play. A play designed to isolate the attacker on a specific defender.

Jump serve. A serve in which the server runs then jumps high to serve. It is difficult but effective because speed is generated and the contact is made from a higher point.

Jungle ball. Any gathering of people playing volleyball who don't use correct techniques.

Key. To discern the opposing team's next play by observing its patterns or habits.

Kill. An attack that results in an immediate point or side out.

Line. The marks that serve as boundaries of a court.

Line shot. A ball spiked along the opponent's sideline that is closest to the hitter and outside the block.

Middle back. A defensive system that uses the middle back player to cover deep spikes.

Middle up. A defensive system that uses the middle back player to cover dinks or short shots.

Mintonette. The original name of the game of volleyball, which was created by William Morgan.

Multiple offense. A system of play that uses various sets, not just outside regular sets.

Offside block. The player at the net on the side that is away from the opponent's attack.

Off-speed hit. A ball that loses power quickly because it was hit with less than usual force.

Off-speed shot. Any ball spiked with less than maximum force but with spin.

On hand. A ball set from the same side as the attacker's favored hand; also called "strong side."

Overhand pass. A pass made with both hands open, controlled by the fingers, with the player's face below the ball.

Overhand serve. A serve in which a player strikes the ball with his or her hand above the shoulder.

Overhead pass. A ball-handling skill in which the player uses both hands simultaneously to contact the ball above the head and to direct it to the intended target.

Pancake. A one-hand floor defensive technique where the player's extended hand slides along the floor palm down while the player dives or extension rolls, so that the ball bounces off the back of the player's hand.

Pass. The first hit, which is aimed at the setter.

Power alley. A cross-court hit that travels away from the spiker to the farthest point of the court.

Ready position. The flexed yet comfortable posture a player assumes before moving to the point of contact.

Roof. To block a spike, usually straight down for a point.

Rotation. The clockwise movement of players around the court and through the serving position following a side out.

Serve. One of the six basic volleyball skills; the serve puts the ball into play.

Set. The tactical skill in which a ball is directed to a point where a player can spike it into the opponent's court.

Setter. The player who makes the set to the attackers.

Side out. Occurs when the receiving team successfully puts the ball away against the serving team, or when the serving team commits an unforced error; the receiving team thus gains the right to serve.

Spike. Also "hit" or "attack"; a ball contacted with force by a player on the offensive team with the intent to terminate the ball on the opponent's floor or off the opponent's blocker.

Sprawl. A technique used to get to a low serve or spike.

Stuff. A ball that is deflected back to the attacking team's floor by the opponent's blockers.

Target area. The area toward which the pass is directed; the setter is released into this area to prepare to set.

Tip. Another term for "dink."

Transition. The term for changing from offense to defense or defense to offense; it must be done quickly and accurately.

Underhand pass. Same as a bump.

Volley. An overhand pass or set.

Wipeoff. An offensive shot that is brushed off the blocker's arms then goes out of bounds.

Zones. A numbering system that designates the placement of a player or the target area of the ball. A common numbering system designates the back right third of the court (the area of the server) as zone 1. Zone 2 is the right front court. Zone 3 is the middle front third of the court. Zone 4 is the left front third. Zone 5 is the left back area and zone 6 is the middle back area.

Summary

1. There are six players on a regulation volleyball team.
2. A game ends at 15 points, but must be won by two points. Thus it would be possible to have a game ending at 21–19, or even 30–28. College and international rules now have a 17 point cap on the game so a game could be won 17–16.

3. A team can score points only when it is serving.
4. When a serving team commits a violation it is a side out and the other team gains the serve.
5. Three contacts (not counting a contact by a blocker) are allowed before the ball must cross the net.
6. The ball can be played with any part of the body on first contact.
7. The rules often change, so the player must keep current on rule updates.

4

Forearm Passing or Bumping

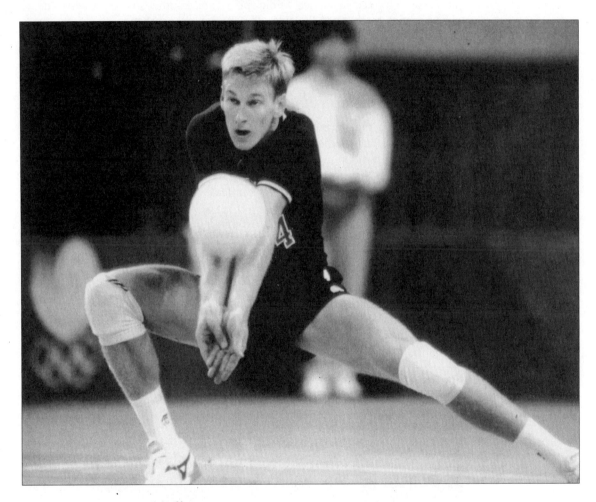

Outline

The term *passing* is used to denote the first contact of a team after the ball has crossed the net on a serve or other type of hit. The pass is directed to the setter. The setter will then set to the attacker.

The *forearm pass* is the most frequently used skill in the game of volleyball. It is, therefore, a very important skill and should be learned first. Without some mastery of this skill, volleyball cannot be played well at any level. The forearm pass is used to receive service, to dig spikes, and in other situations when the player cannot get in a good position to pass the ball overhand.

The forearm pass, or *bump*, should be hit high enough and accurately enough to allow the setter time to make a perfect set to the attacker.

Making the Pass

Where possible, the player should move the body in line with the flight of the ball so that the ball can be played forward of the body and at the body's mid-line. Slide to a position in front of the ball. Do not cross your legs when moving sideways unless there is a long distance to be covered. Also remember to keep your feet on the ground. Never leave your feet to make a pass—the legs act as shock absorbers, not propellants.

Try to keep your body movement to a minimum, since there is really very little time to move if the serve is hard or you are playing a spiked ball. Because of the lower net in women's leagues, women may need a lower stance than men because the ball can come in at a sharper angle.

The passer should play the ball low. Your knees should be flexed with the feet slightly wider than shoulder width apart. Your feet should be staggered with your right foot forward. It is possible when passing at an angle for the foot closest to the direction of the pass to be slightly forward. For example, if the

Starting position	**Side view of receiving position**
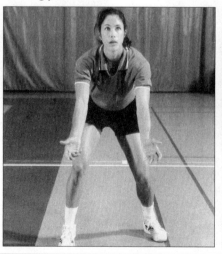	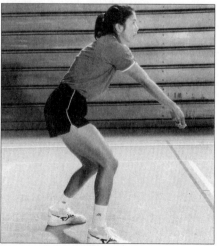

a.

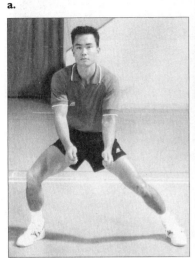

b.

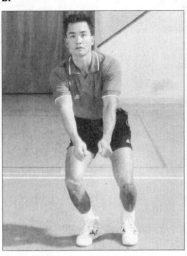

c.

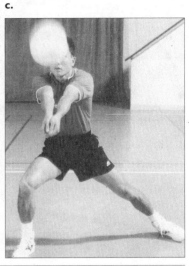

**a. Passer moving laterally to ball;
b. Passer not crossing legs during movement;
c. Re-establishing wide base with right foot forward**

passer is on the outside edge of the court and is directing the pass forward and toward the center, the outside foot can be back to make it easier for the passer to aim the pass back into the court by shifting the weight or striding toward the target area.

Your back should be bent slightly forward and your head should be slightly down. With your head down, your eyes can follow the ball almost to the point of contact on your forearms. With your weight carried forward, you should feel more weight on your toes, particularly on your inside toes.

To make the *passing platform*, your arms should be straight, elbows locked, the heels of your hands (near the wrist) touching. Both hands will be pointing

**a. Close up forearm platform with contact points;
b. Ball on contact points**

a.

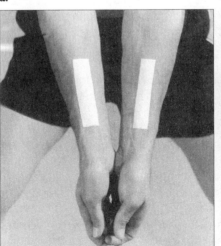

b.

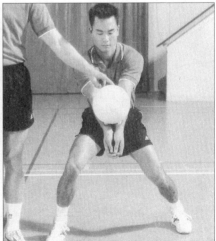

Checklist for the Pass

1. Set your feet wider than your shoulders with your right foot forward.
2. Your back should be bent forward and your head should be down with your eyes focused on the ball.
3. Your knees should be bent to whatever angle is necessary to be able to play the ball between your waist and the knees.
4. With your elbows locked and your hands interlocking and with the heels of your hands touching and pointed downward, gently guide the ball toward the target area. The angle of your arms to the floor will determine the arc of the ball.
5. Set the angle of your platform prior to contacting the ball.
6. Your body weight should shift forward toward the target as the ball is contacted. This assists in achieving the proper trajectory.

toward the floor so that the fleshy part of your forearms is exposed. Your radius bone (the long bone from the elbow to the thumb side of the wrist) is rotated outward so that the ball will not contact it. This gives you a wider platform area with which to control the ball. The ball should be contacted two to six inches above your wrists.

The key to making a flat platform with the forearms is to have the bases of your hands touching and even—neither one higher than the other. The fingers are commonly overlapped, but they may be slightly interlocked or even separated from each other as long as your arms do not break apart. Your fingers should not form a fist.

Rather than swinging at the ball, use your arms as a platform so that the ball will rebound in the proper direction and with the desired arc. It is important to "set the angle" of the platform prior to contacting the ball. Think soft—softly shovel and guide the ball into your target area. The harder the spike or serve is hit at you, the more you must absorb the speed of the ball while making the pass.

Your body and arms will move slightly forward as the pass, or bump, is made. The ball should be contacted at a height between your waist and your knees.

The angle of your arms from your shoulders will determine the arc of the ball. It is a law of physics that the angle of incidence equals the angle of refraction. So if a ball is coming at a 30-degree angle to the lower part of your arm, it will leave at a 30-degree angle to the upper part of your arm. With practice you will begin to feel the proper angle of your arms for the desired arc of the pass. Generally, an angle of approximately 45 degrees to the floor will be best.

As the pass is made, shift your weight in the direction of the target. A shuffle step with your lead foot can also assist the ball in the direction of the target.

Front view of passing posture with contact points visible

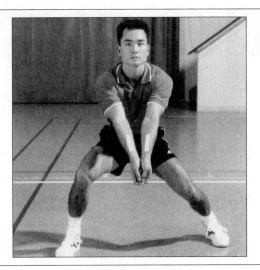

The *height* of the pass is the most difficult thing to control. A pass that is too high may cause problems for the attacker and give the defense time to get set. Generally, a pass should follow an arc high enough to allow the setter to get into position and to set the ball. The target area should be about two and one-half feet from the net.

Anticipate your play by being aware of your position on the court and where your target area will be. Then concentrate on the opponent's server—always expecting the ball to come to you. Be "fast to the ball" once you have determined the direction of the serve or spike. It is important to get "behind" the ball quickly rather than "under" the ball quickly.

Analyze the server's style. Does the server use a top spin serve or a jump serve that will dive quickly after it crosses the net? If so, position yourself closer

a. Close up forearm platform with contact points; b. Ball on contact points

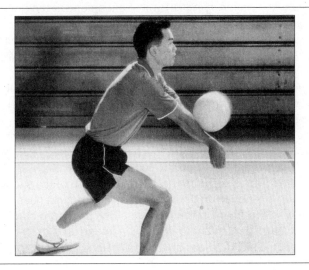

Checklist for Common Errors in Passing

1. Establishing your hitting platform too late
2. Making the platform too close to your body
3. Bending or swinging your platform
4. Contacting the ball too low on your forearms or wrists

to the net to be able to play the dropping ball. Does the server like to serve down the line or cross-court? Position yourself to take away the expected serve.

Concentration is a major factor. Your eyes must be on the person hitting the ball—the server or spiker. The point of contact and the follow-through will give you an idea of the direction and speed of the ball. Since it takes about half a second for an elite volleyball player to see the ball and react with the arms, you can understand why it is so important to concentrate on the hitter instead of the ball and save perhaps a fraction of a second in reaction time. Most beginners wait until they see the ball in flight before they begin to make their preparation for the pass.

Types of Passes

The *pass off the serve* is difficult because the serve is generally coming hard and may be coming with a spin, or, in the case of a flat serve, it may move in an unpredictable way. The one advantage for the receiver is that he or she has more time to prepare for this pass than when playing a spiked ball.

A *pass to a stationary setter* is most often done at the lower levels of play. This is relatively easy to do because the target is stationary.

A *pass to a moving setter* who is switching positions occurs at every level of play. The pass must be made to the target area into which the setter will move and slightly in front of the setter.

A *pass directly to a front court setter/attacker* is occasionally done at the elite level of play to reduce the effectiveness of a block. The passer passes directly to the setter/attacker, who may then spike the ball.

The *attacking pass* is occasionally used when the passer notes a wide opening in the defensive alignment. Such a situation may occur when one or more players have been forced off the court to play a ball.

A *lateral pass* is sometimes required. Because of the spontaneous nature of the game, it is not always possible to make a perfect pass from the midline of the body. When the ball is to the side of the passer and the passer is unable to pass the ball from the body's midline, a lateral pass must be attempted. The player should step to a position with a trailing foot, allowing a weight shift to

**Extended stride to
receive short ball**

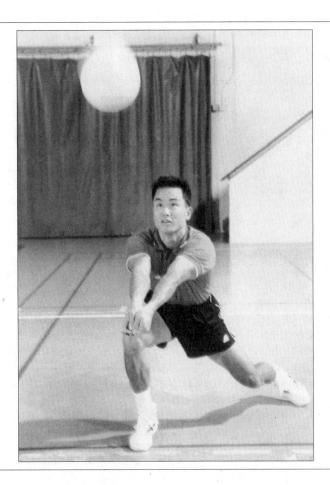

**Preparing for lateral
pass**

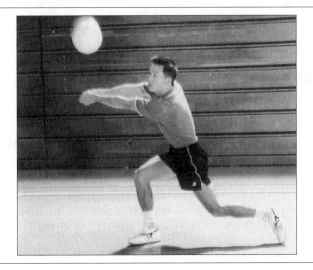

Executing lateral pass

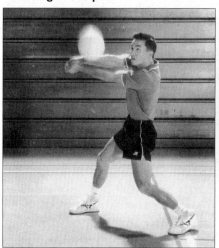

Passing a high ball

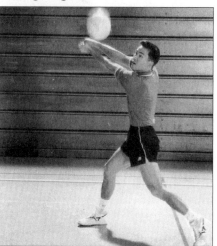

occur. The ball should still be played before it crosses the plane of the body. Because the ball is being played outside of the midline of the body, it must be played farther in front of the body to ensure the proper angle required to complete the pass.

In the lateral pass the forearm platform is maintained as in a regular pass, but the arms are extended to the side of the body. The platform will be angled so that the ball can be directed from the contact point at the side of the body toward the target area. This is done by lifting the arm farthest from the target and tilting the platform forward toward the target.

The *highball pass* is necessary when the ball cannot be played low. It can be done with open hands, as in a set (see Chapter 6), or with a reverse forearm pass. However, it is difficult to play a hard-hit ball with open hands and not be called for a "double contact" or for "holding" it.

The *reverse forearm pass* is executed when the ball is at chest height or higher. The passer flexes the knees if necessary so that the pass can be taken at head height. The hands and forearms are kept in the same relative position as in a low pass, but the elbows are at about head height and pointed forward. The ball is contacted on the back of the forearms on the ulnar bone (the bone that is on the same side of the arm as the little finger) and angled upward and toward the target area.

Practice for passing is best done by receiving serves. While beginning drills will be done with one person tossing the ball softly to the passer, realistic game drills will be done by returning serves.

When *receiving the serve*, remember that while the ball will travel more slowly than a spiked ball, it will often change directions because of the buildup of air pressure in front of the ball. It may move up, down, or to the side. In fact, it may make several such movements during the flight from the server.

Checklist for Learning Progression

Beginner skills

1. Toss to the passer
2. Pass to a stationary target/setter
3. Pass from a serve

Intermediate skills

4. Lateral pass (outside midline of body)
5. High ball pass (above midline of body)
6. Pass to a moving setter

Advanced skills

7. Low trajectory pass
8. Pass to setter/attacker

Watch the server to determine the angle of the follow-through and the action of the wrist to be able to get the jump on the ball.

Front-row players should not play balls that are above waist level. Leave them for the back-court players. If the ball is played by a front-row player, the back-row players must back up the play in case the ball is not passed perfectly. Back-row players should play 60 to 70 percent of the balls.

Drills

1. (Pairs) Partners pass to each other.
2. (Pairs) Each partner gets two hits in a row—a bump to oneself, then a bump back to the partner. Variations include:
   a. Bump to self, then bump to partner.
   b. Bump to self, make a quarter turn, then bump to partner.
   c. Bump to self, make a half turn, then bump to partner.
   d. Bump to self, make a full turn, then bump to partner.
3. (Pairs) Each partner gets three hits in succession. Variations include:
   a. Bump to self, squat and make an overhand pass (set) to self, then bump to partner.
   b. Bump to self, squat and bump to self, bump to partner.
   c. (Intermediate and advanced players) Bump to self, do a forward roll, bump to self again, then bump to partner.

Triangle passing:
The three players forming the triangle can rotate on time or criteria established by the instructor.

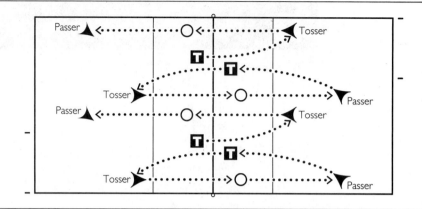

Partner passing

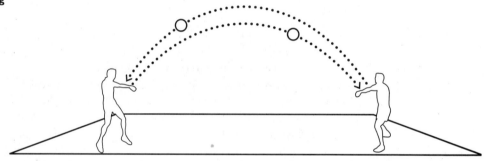

Pass to self, pass to partner

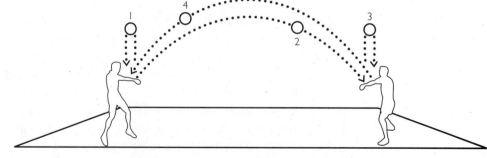

Pass to self, 1/4 turn, pass to partner

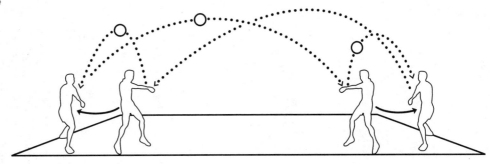

Pass to self, 1/2 turn, pass to partner

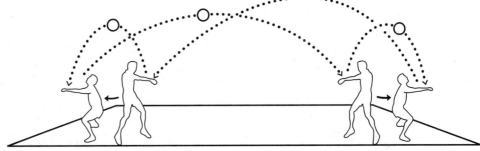

Pass to self, full turn, pass to partner

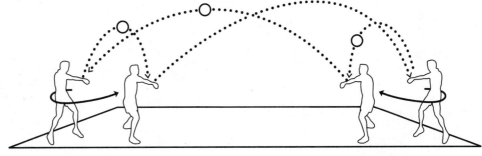

**Pass, squat, pass,
pass to partner**

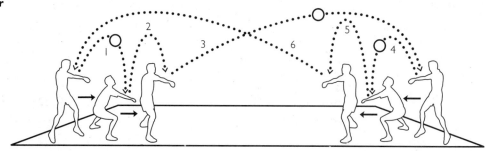

Pass, pass, pass

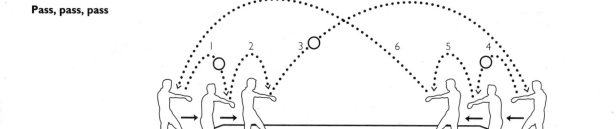

Team-serve-receive:
Players can rotate
on time or criteria
designed by the
instructor. The
instructor should
ensure some degree
of success.

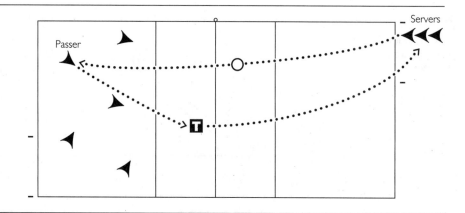

4. (Pairs) Partner alternates throwing the ball to the passer—at different heights, different directions (right and left), and different speeds—throwing harder as the player becomes more adept at passing.

5. (Pairs or teams) One side serves while the receivers make passes to a target or to a setter.

6. As soon as possible, make all passes from a ball coming from the other side of the net—first thrown, then served, then spiked.

Summary

1. Passing the ball is the primary skill necessary for success in volleyball.

2. The pass is used to get the ball in play after the opponents have served or have returned the ball.

3. The pass is made from below waist level with the arms extended.

4. The passer must concentrate on the ball from the time it leaves the hand of the server or attacker.

5 *The Serve*

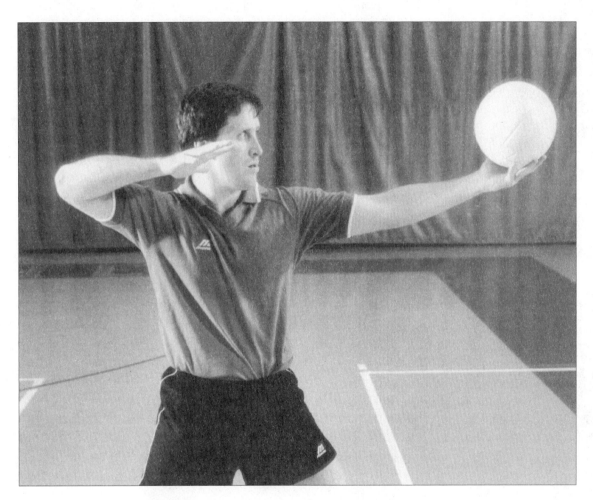

Outline

The serve is obviously an integral part of a volleyball match. A highly effective serve will score an outright winner—an ace. Even if it is not an outright winner, a serve can still put the opponents in a weaker position by forcing an errant pass and possibly a weak set. The best method of derailing a potent offense is to deliver a tough serve and force them into a slower or less desirable option of attack.

There are several types of serves. Top players may master several, but few players master them all. For beginners, the most important factors in serving are speed and accuracy. The first goal is to get the ball into the court with speed; the next concern is to maneuver the ball to the defense's weakness.

The rules require that the server remain behind the end line until the ball is contacted. The server must serve the ball from within three meters of the right sideline. If the server serves from too wide a position or steps on the line before the ball leaves his or her hand, it is considered a fault and the serve is lost.

The Underhand Serve

The *underhand serve* can be extremely effective at the beginning level. Since it is easy to learn it has a greater chance of achieving the 90 percent accuracy rate that is the goal for beginning-level players.

The *stance* begins by facing the target, then taking a stride forward with the leg on the nonserving side. Your feet should be about shoulder-width apart.

Starting posture for underhand serve

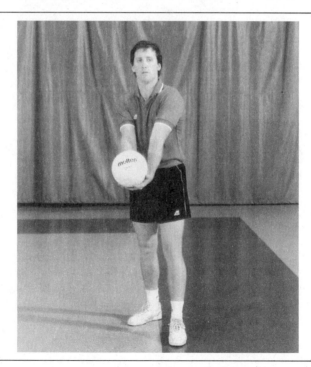

Serving arm drawn back

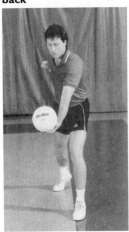

Ball lift and stride

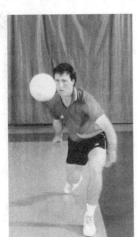

Arm swing prior to contact

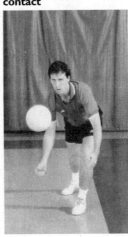

Contacting the ball

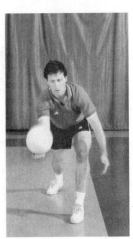

Your forward foot should face the direction of the serve, and your knees should be slightly flexed. Your foot cannot touch the line. Most players serve from two to ten feet behind the back line.

The *serving action* starts with the ball in your nonserving hand (the left hand for right-handed servers). The ball is held with the palm up, in front and outside of the serving-side hip. The ball is tossed straight up just a few inches from the nonserving hand. (Hitting directly from the hand is illegal.)

Swing your hitting arm backward as you shift your weight to your rear foot and turn your shoulders away from the net with the backswing. Your weight then shifts forward and your hips and shoulders rotate toward the target. Swing your arm forward and contact the ball with the heel of your hand and a stiff wrist or a fist. (The stiff wrist limits the amount of spin on the ball.) The ball is

Side view of stride

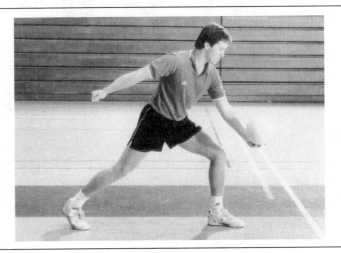

contacted below the center. Keep your eyes on the ball throughout the serve. Your arm follows through toward the target and you move into the court, ready to take up your assigned defensive position.

A high underhand serve may be quite difficult for the receivers to play. Indoors, the ball may move unexpectedly because of the buildup of air pressure under the ball. Outdoors, the ball may be carried by the wind, which will alter its trajectory and make it hard to handle. If it is sunny and the opponents are facing the sun, the ball may be played so that it is hidden in the sun.

The Overhand Serve

There are several types of overhand serves: floaters, spins, and jumps. Each has a unique technical form.

For all types of overhand serves, your *starting position* is facing the net with your feet shoulder-width apart and under your shoulders. For right-handed servers, the left foot will be forward in a comfortable stance. The ball is held in both hands at about chest to shoulder height. The nonserving hand is under the ball while the serving hand rests on top.

The *backswing* is like a catcher's throw rather than a full-arm swing. Your elbow is drawn back and remains above your shoulder. As you draw your arm back, your shoulder and hips rotate away from the net. At or near the end of this action, toss the ball up about two feet high and about 12 to 18 inches in front of your hitting shoulder. A low, accurate toss helps the serve to be efficient.

The *stride* with the nonhitting side leg starts the serving action. As you step forward, shift your weight to your forward foot and turn your hips and shoulders toward the net. Your hitting arm closely follows in a forward action.

Starting posture for float serve

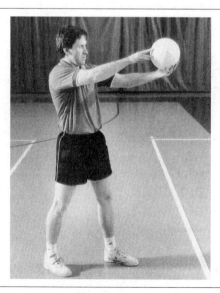

Checklist for the Overhand Serve

1. *Starting position.* Feet pointing nearly at target, upper body 45 degrees from target.
2. *Backswing.* Short.
3. *Toss.* In front of head, farther back if serving very high.
4. *Stride.* Short stride and weight shifted forward.
5. *Contact.* More under the ball for a high serve; more behind for low serve.
6. *Follow-through.* At the target.

The *elbow leads the hand and arm* as the hitting arm comes forward. Your shoulder comes forward, then your elbow extends, then the wrist follows through. Contact the ball just above head height and in front of your hitting shoulder.

The wrist remains stiff and your hand is open to offer the largest surface area possible. The wrist should not turn, but should direct your hand toward the serving target.

The *two-count toss* is often valuable for beginners because it can give them more power. In this movement your striking-side leg steps forward (the right leg for right-handed servers). Draw your striking hand back as you make your first step.

Backswing:
a. Drawing the serving elbow and hand back;
b. Start of arm swing, with elbow lead and ball placement

a.

b.

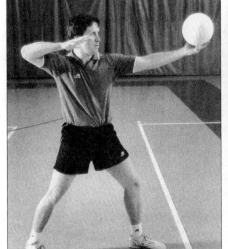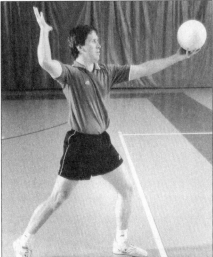

Arm position just prior to contact

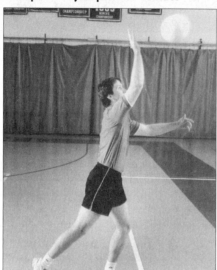

Post–ball contact showing open firm hand

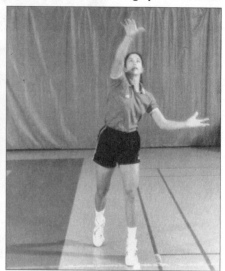

The toss is made as you start your second step. As your weight is transferred to the nonstriking-side foot (the left foot for right-handers), move your arm forward and strike the ball.

Contact the ball with the palm of your hand. The trajectory of the ball should be nearly flat. A high-trajectory overhand serve is no more effective than an underhand serve.

The *follow-through* is toward the target. As your arm follows through, move into the court to take up your assigned position.

The Float Serve

The *float* serve is the most commonly used serve at elite levels of play in the United States. It is a nonspinning ball that moves with existing air currents. To perform a float serve, begin with the same stance as the underhand serve. Generally, you should take a position from two to ten feet behind the back line. Your nonserving leg is forward and your feet are about shoulder-width apart.

Hold the ball with your palm up and at about chest level or higher. Toss the ball from an area in front of your hitting shoulder with your nonserving hand. It should be two to three feet high and just in front of your hitting-side shoulder. Keep your eyes on the ball throughout the serve. Because the valve of the ball makes that area of the ball heavier, the ball may drift to the side of the valve; this theory has been advanced for years, but it has not actually been proven.

Swing your hitting arm back as you shift your weight to your rear foot. Then move your weight forward and swing through with your hips, then your shoulders. Your arm follows as in a baseball throw. Contact the ball in the middle of

Checklist for the Float Serve

1. Stand back from the back line facing the court.
2. Set the valve stem where you want it.
3. Toss the ball in front of the hitting shoulder and two to three feet high—with no spin.
4. Hit into the back of the ball.
5. Limit the follow-through.
6. Get back into defense.

the back of the ball with an open hand; the contact point is slightly higher than your head. The primary impact is with the heel of your hand. Your wrist should be locked.

There is little follow-through because the ball is punched. (Note, however, that a player who is not very strong may have to follow through.) After serving, the player moves into the court to play defense.

A hard float serve is struck hard on the middle of the ball. It moves faster and is lower than the regular float serve.

Two-step serve:
a. Second and final step of two-step serve;
b. Side view of two step float serve showing first of two steps

a.
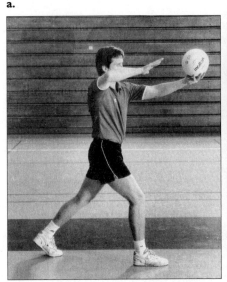

b.
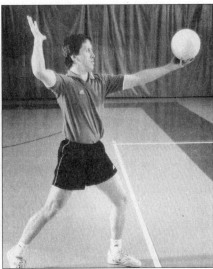

Initial posture for top-spin serve

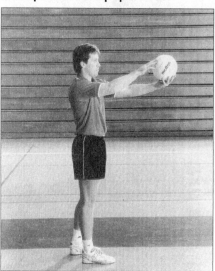

Ball lift and back arch

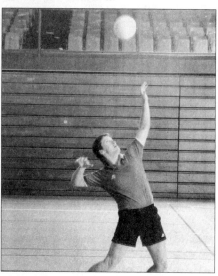

The Top-Spin Serve

The *top-spin serve* is effective because it allows for a fairly powerful serve with relative accuracy. With the top-spin, the server takes a position much the same as for a tennis serve. The ball is tossed up as the hitting shoulder rotates away from the ball.

The ball is tossed higher than for a floater to allow the player to hit the underside of the ball (about 30 degrees below the center of the back of the

Arm extension and contact point, snapping the wrist to put top spin on ball

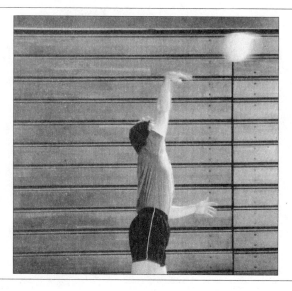

ball), then drive the hand over the top of the ball with a snap of the wrist.

As a variation, your hand can follow through to either side of the ball, causing a side spin. This can be especially effective when you are playing outside with a cross-wind. The ball can be spun so that the wind's role in pushing the ball is greatly increased.

The Jump Serve

The *jump serve* can be highly effective, but it is rather risky. Because of all the variables involved (the run, jump, and wrist action), accuracy is reduced.

Jump serve:
a. Initial posture for jump serve; b. First step of approach, c. Ball placement (lift) and start of jump; d. Full lift and jump just prior to contact; e. Post contact position with follow-through

a.
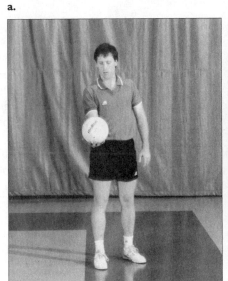

b.
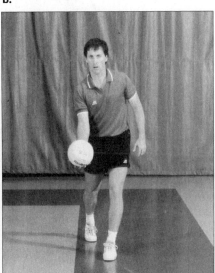

c.
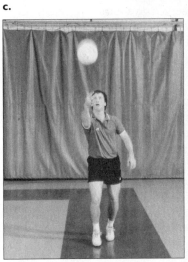

d.
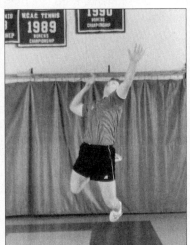

e.
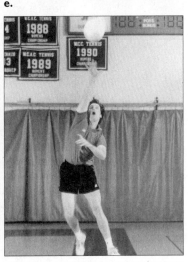

Checklist of Common Errors in Serving

1. Having a problem in timing the serving action such as bringing your arm through before you shift your weight or turned your hips. This type of error is often made by people who have not had much experience in throwing.
2. Taking too short a stride to get an effective weight shift.
3. Bringing the arm through too low in the forward swing.
4. Not serving fast enough (arm action too slow).
5. Having the wrist too loose on contact with the ball.
6. Failing to hit the center of the ball.

The start of the serve is the same as an approach for a spike. For a right-handed server, the four-step approach would be right, left, right, close, jump. The three-step approach would start with the left leg. The toss is made prior to the "step, close" portion of the approach so that the ball can be contacted at the peak of the jump and slightly ahead of the body. The toss can be made with one or two hands.

As with the spike, the hand and wrist snaps over the top to achieve power and control. Most players toss the ball so that their momentum actually carries them over the end line of the court. This is legal as long as the ball is contacted prior to landing. The momentum of the approach and the jump is transferred to the ball, greatly increasing the arm power and ball speed.

As with the top-spin serve, the action of the wrist can make the ball spin sideways, making it an even tougher serve. The speed and spin of the ball make it very difficult to play at the lower levels of volleyball, but at the elite level the skill of the passers reduces the serve's effectiveness because they can predict where the ball will land. Hard spinning serves give a true trajectory, as opposed to the floater serve, which moves in an unpredictable direction.

Other Considerations

The *serving areas* (zones 1 through 6) may be targeted by the coach in high levels of play. At lower levels, the players should simply be aware that they should have a specific target to which to serve. Using the whole court as the target is appropriate only for the very beginning-level player.

Varying the trajectories is another way to complicate the opponents' passing. By beginning with high, deep serves to force the passers to align deeper into their court, the server can open up the front area for shorter-diving top-spin serves.

Serving area

Service target areas

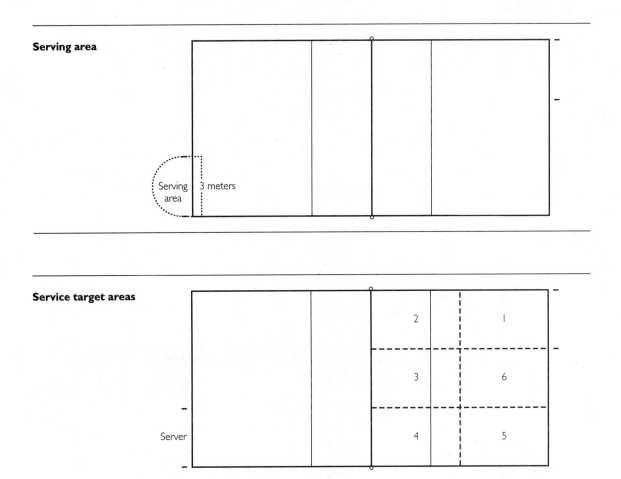

It is important for passers to avoid getting into a rhythm of playing balls of the same speed and trajectory. The good server will vary serves to prevent receivers from discovering a predictable pattern.

Concentration and *ritual* are the final considerations for serving. By developing a ritual or procedure to use before each serve, you can prepare your body for the relatively simple motor action of the serve. This also helps you relax and concentrate.

For example, a simple ritual might be to simply bounce the ball once or twice; a more complicated ritual might be to close your eyes, take three deep breaths to relax, then put the middle finger of your tossing hand on the valve.

High trajectory serve

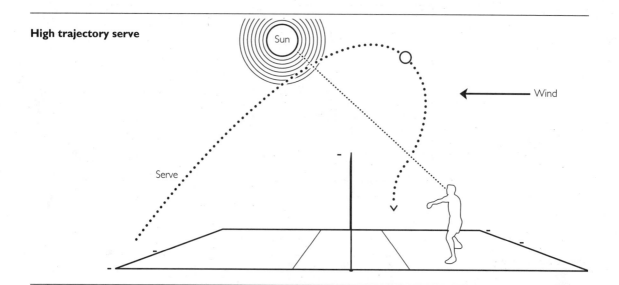

Sun

Wind

Serve

Checklist for Server's Priorities

1. Be consistent by getting nearly every serve into the court.
2. Serve to the proper target area—the weak player or the vulnerable area (rear corners or seams between the players).
3. Higher-level players should do something special to the serve—increased speed, a tricky spin, or a lack of spin.

Strategies for Serving

- Always know your target area and the type of serve you want to hit before beginning your service action.
- Identify the weakest serve returner on the opposing team before the game, or find out quickly who it is. A substitute who has just entered the game may be a good target, because he or she may not be warmed up.
- The weakest areas in a defense are usually the deep corners, the side lines, the short middle area, and the seams between players.
- When serving a seam, have the valve facing in the direction of the weaker player.
- Serve to a player who has just mishandled a serve.
- Serving away from the strongest spiker makes passing more difficult for the opposition.

- Occasionally serve into the setter's path as he or she moves from the back court to the forecourt.
- Vary the targets as your opponents adjust their serve receive.
- The primary concern of the server is to get the ball over the net and in play.

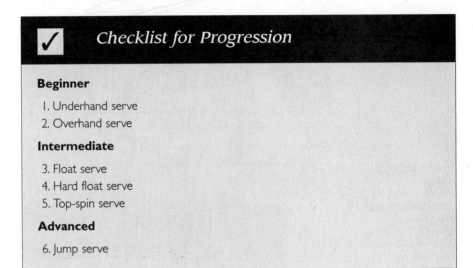

✓   *Checklist for Progression*

Beginner

1. Underhand serve
2. Overhand serve

Intermediate

3. Float serve
4. Hard float serve
5. Top-spin serve

Advanced

6. Jump serve

Drills

Serving practices should be distributed throughout the practice session rather than done as one long segment during the practice.

1. *Partner serving.* Servers at each end of the court serve into the opposite court.
2. *Target serving.* Set up targets, people, or "Bozos" (air-filled, bottom-weighted, pop-up simulated clowns). Serve to hit the target.

Partner serving

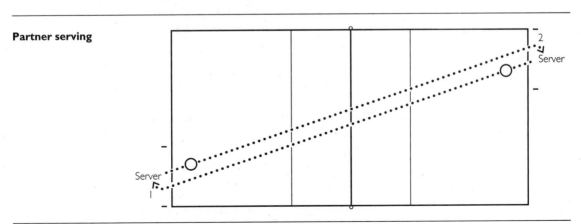

Target serving

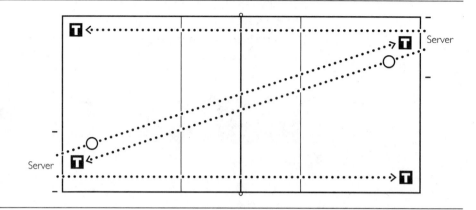

4 versus 2 triangle serving:
To score a point the passer must pass four perfect passes consecutively. The server scores when the passer fails to pass perfectly two consecutive times. The scoring criteria can be adjusted to fit the level of play.

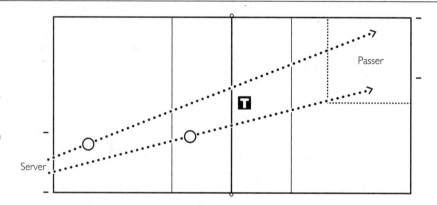

3. *Four-two triangle serving.* One server versus two passers and a setter. Passers get one point if they make four consecutive good passes. The server gets a point if he or she makes two good serves that cannot be played.

4. *Pressure serving.* The whole team must serve a series of predetermined serves before leaving practice.

Summary

1. When you are learning to serve, do not sacrifice speed for accuracy.

2. Your elbow should be kept high while serving.

3. There are several types of serves: underhand, overhand, spin serves, floaters, jump serves.

4. The server should have a clear idea of where to direct a serve by identifying the weak area of the defense or the weak player in the defense.

6

Setting and the Overhand Pass

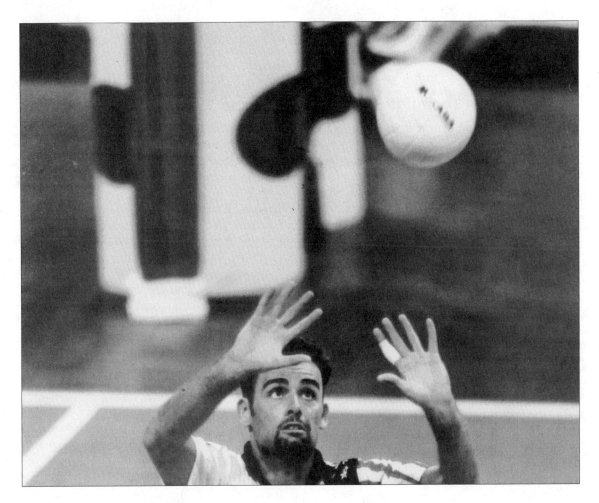

Outline

The set is generally an overhand pass that is directed to the point where the attacker can best hit it for a kill. The setter is expected to make a perfect set to the attacker so that the attacker can make the most effective play possible. Because passers often make poor passes, the setter should be a gifted athlete who is capable of running down errant passes.

The overhand pass should be used whenever possible (except on serve reception and when digging), because it is a very accurate method of passing the ball. It can be legally used on any shot, but it is very difficult to execute without making a double contact if the ball is coming fast, as in a serve or spike.

Techniques of the Overhand Pass

Get behind the ball as quickly as possible. Watch the passer in order to get an early tip on the direction and height of the pass. If you can't be standing in one spot when the pass arrives, at least try to stop your body by shuffling to the spot, and stop momentarily even though your momentum is moving you. It is best not to set while running.

Drawing the hands to the setting position is done by bringing the hands quickly upward along the front of the body to a position directly above the upturned forehead. Beginners often bring their hands away from the body. This causes the setter to make contact with the ball in different areas above the forehead.

The hands are *shaped* by spreading the fingers and cupping them. They should be formed so that they will cup the ball when it contacts them. When ready to contact the ball, the index fingers and thumbs should form a triangle. The tips of the thumbs should be one to three inches apart and the tips of the

Overhand pass:
a. In position to set;
b. Drawing up of the hands; c. Hands drawn and shaped; d. Side view of hands drawn and shaped

a. b. c. d.

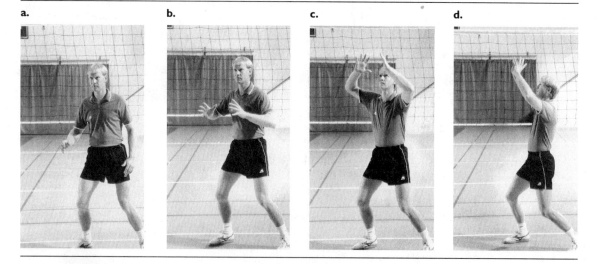

Front and back views of hands forming triangle

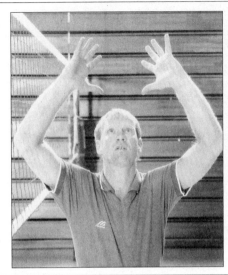 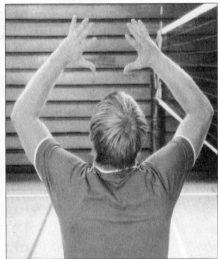

index fingers should be two to four inches apart. (This varies with the size of the hands; players with smaller hands should hold them farther apart.) The thumbs should point slightly back toward the forehead.

The actual point of contact will be the pads of the fingers and thumbs—about an inch back from the fingertips. All of the fingers should touch the ball, but most of the pressure will be felt on the thumbs and forefingers. The outside fingers will help to control the ball.

Front and back views of triangle with ball

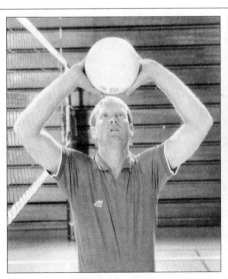 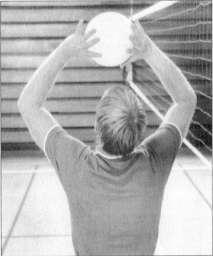

✓ Checklist for the Overhand Set

1. The feet should be slightly staggered and about shoulder-width apart, with the right foot forward.
2. The body should be bent slightly forward.
3. The upper arms should be parallel with the floor.
4. The hands should be in front of and above the upturned forehead.
5. The hands should be shaped for the ball and the wrists turned back so that the thumbs point toward the forehead.
6. All the fingers should touch the ball on the finger pads.
7. Face the target with the shoulders and head and, if possible, the feet.
8. Follow through by extending the body and arms in the direction of the arc that is desired for the ball to follow.

The *fingers* should be somewhat rigid, yet flexible. They should not be so stiff that the ball rebounds immediately nor so relaxed that the ball settles into the hands and is illegally caught.

The *wrists and forearms* act as shock absorbers, because they absorb the weight and force of the ball then launch it again into flight. The wrists should be in a comfortable, hyperextended (bent toward the back of the forearms) position as the ball approaches. The arms, not the wrists, supply the power. Because of this, forearm strength is necessary for good setting.

The *elbows* should beset apart slightly wider than the shoulders. The elbows are prime power sources for the set. The primary power comes from the exten-

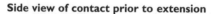

Side view of contact prior to extension   **Arm extension**

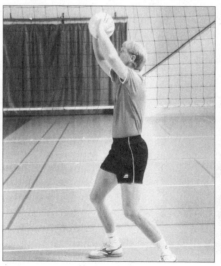
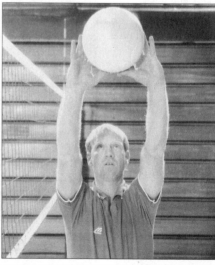

a. Hand and arm follow-through;
b. Stepping away from the net to pursue a pass that is away from the net

a.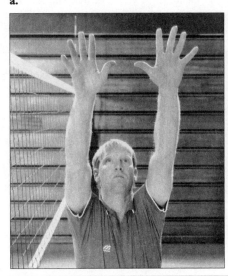

b.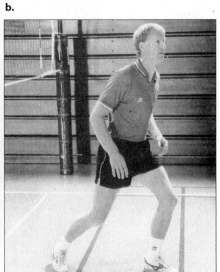

sion of the elbows, not the flexion of the wrists. Beginners often use wrist action, which is likely to cause errant passes. The job of the wrists is to control the ball as the extension of the elbows supplies the power.

The power from the elbows must be equal from each elbow or the ball will not fly true. For example, too much power from the right arm will make the ball move to the left of the setter. When the player sets, both arms should be fully extended to ensure an even release.

a. The second step of pursuit; b. Hands drawn and shaped with feet squared to left front attack position

a.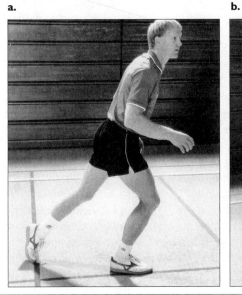

b.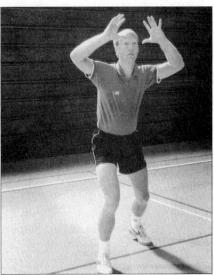

Ball contact prior to extension

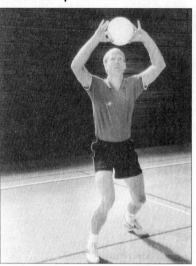

Extension and follow-through

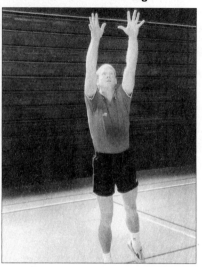

The *shoulders* are essential in aiming the set. They should be aimed directly at the target area. If they are not correctly positioned the ball may be "carried," resulting in a foul. For example, if the target is to the right of the setter and the shoulders are not squared to the target, the left hand will probably stay on the ball longer than the right hand and a "carry" will result. Also, such a set cannot be controlled as well as one in which both arms supply equal impetus to the ball. Not properly squaring the shoulders and feet toward the target area is the most common error in setting.

Leg flexion is important, especially for younger players who may not have the upper body strength to set with ball without leg motion. Beginning players are encouraged to use a great deal of knee flexion when setting. This is true whether the set is long and high or short and low. Every setting motion should be uniform to reduce the ability of the smarter opponents to predict the kind of set you will make. However, on long sets it is essential to use leg power; in fact, it is not uncommon to see elite players leave their feet as they follow through on long sets. This indicates the considerable amount of leg power they were exerting—even if their legs were not greatly flexed, their ankle muscles helped provide great power.

Some advanced players set the ball with their legs straight, but their upper body strength compensates for this. They do this so that the blockers aren't able to "key" on the amount of knee flexion that they use and thereby tell whether the set will be long or short. If the blocker reads the setter correctly he or she will be able to anticipate where the ball will go even before it leaves the setter's hands. So at the higher levels of play, perfection and deception are desired.

If at all possible, the set should be made with an overhand pass. This requires the setter to bend greatly at the knees while maintaining the hands high in order to accurately set balls that have been passed low.

Checklist for Common Errors in Setting

1. Getting to the ball too late.
2. Failing to take the ball at the same contact point (above the forehead) each time.
3. Getting the hands up too late.
4. Having the thumbs forward rather than shaped to the ball.
5. Failure to extend to a full reach during the follow-through.

Foot positioning is as important as shoulder positioning. For most people the feet should be shoulder-width apart, with the right foot forward for better stability. The feet should be pointing at the target area during the setting motion unless the set is an overhead or back set. (Many beginners face the passer rather than the attacker when setting; this is wrong.) However, the feet and shoulders will open toward the passer as the ball is received, then they are rotated back (squared) to the target as the set is made.

Some teachers prefer that the foot nearest the net be forward in order to reduce the chance of the set being made too close to the net. The authors prefer that every fundamental be the same in order to reduce errors. They therefore believe in having the same foot forward on all sets whether made facing the right or the left.

The *contact point* is above the forehead. The setter should watch the ball through the opening between the thumbs and index fingers. The ball is taken "on" (above) the forehead.

The *follow-through* is very important for accuracy and control. The ball will always go in the direction that it is aimed. If it doesn't go where you desire, you did not aim it there or follow through correctly. The wrists and arms should continue in the direction of the set. Always extend your body through the ball as you follow through.

Varying Types of Sets

Off passes are passes that pull the setter away from the target area. The setter should move past the ball then turn the body back toward where the attacker will hit. Beginners often merely get to the ball, then have problems setting the ball to the outside. They are likely to throw the ball because they are not squared to the direction of the set.

The setter must get the feet beyond the ball, get set facing the target, then shift the weight forward into the set. If the player does not get beyond the ball, it is likely to fall short of the target.

The *back set* (reverse set) allows the setter to deceive the blockers by using the entire length of the net, no matter which way he or she is facing. The back

Jump set:
a. Start of jump for jump set; b. Drawing the hands for jump set; c. Jumping to the ball with hands shaped

a.   b.   c.

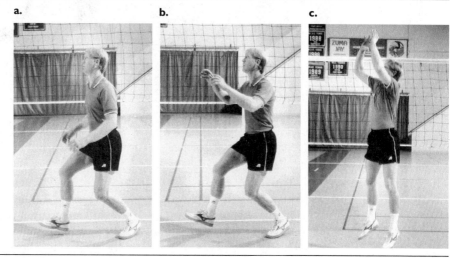

set should look just like the front set so that the blockers are not able to detect where the set will be targeted. However, the back will be slightly arched and the head will be back so that the arms can direct the ball to the rear and the setter can watch the flight of the ball during the follow-through.

The back set is contacted in the same place as the front set. A common error is that the setter will place the hands lower for a front set and higher for a back set. Another error is running too far under the ball when making the reverse set.

It should be noted that when there is an errant pass, a ball hit high into the net will generally rebound downward, while ball hit into the low part of the net will usually rebound outward. The exact angle of the ball coming off the net is

Contact on the jump set

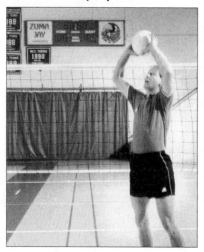

Jump set extension and follow-through

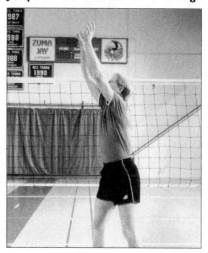

Arm and hand position for one-handed set

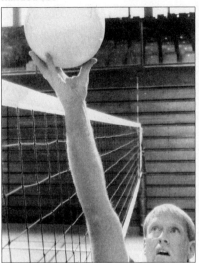

Executing the one-handed set

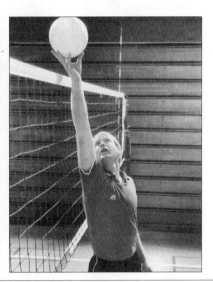

determined by its speed, the angle at which it hit the net, and the place on the net where it hit.

The setter must note all of the variables listed above, then estimate where the netted ball will go. The setter should then adjust accordingly and drop down as low as possible to play the ball.

The *underhand set* is used as a save technique when it is not possible to set with an overhand pass. It is the same as a bump pass, except that the ball should be placed in an area where the spiker can hit the ball.

The *running set* is a "save" technique used when a ball is passed so poorly that the setter does not have time to get into position and stop. Even in the running set the setter must square to the target area.

The *jump set* is a valuable technique to use at intermediate and advanced levels of play. By jump setting, players can increase their effective range and save many balls that might have been unplayable. They can also stop a high pass that might otherwise have traveled over the net without an attacker hitting it. Jump setting is also a way of quickening the attack and allowing the setter to become a potential offensive threat when in the front row by occasionally attacking from the jump rather than making the expected set.

When positioning for the jump set, the setter should move as soon as possible to a position one step away from where the ball will come down from the pass. The last step allows the player to collect his or her body for a two-foot takeoff, and also gives the setter time to get the hands in the setting position while jumping for the ball.

The jump set requires you to jump as if you were spiking while bringing your hands to the setting position. Time your jump so that the ball is contacted just before the top of the jump. Be sure that your body is facing the direction that you wish the set to travel. If the set is a long one, the follow-through of the arms is very important because there can be no additional power from the legs.

A *backward jump set* is executed using the same techniques as explained for the back set, but is done at the top of the jump.

A *one-handed jump set* is an advanced technique that can be used to save a ball that might otherwise go over the net when the pass is too long. Jump as if you were going to spike the ball, but reach up with your hand closest to the net and, with the fingers spread and stiff and the palm of your hand facing back into your court, make a quick, short contact and direct the ball toward the attacker. The thumb and index finger should be closer together than on a normal set, and the arm and wrist are relatively straight. The power comes from a quick poke or stab of the fingers.

Quick sets are another way of fooling the block. All movements of the setter are kept the same, but the contact is quicker and softer without much follow-through. The primary power comes from the hands and fingers.

The quick set is generally short. It should be set far enough away from the net so that the blockers cannot intercept it, and it should be high enough so that the attacker can contact it at the highest point possible. The setter should be in a position to see the ball and the attacking arm of the quick hitter.

Once the quick set has been established, a crossing action of two hitters can be played. One attacker can move into the position necessary to play the shorter, "quick" set. A second attacker can move in another direction ready to take the higher "play" set. This can confuse the blockers, who must move to stop the quick set then move again to stop the play set.

The *play set in a crossing action* should be slightly beyond and behind the quick hitter to allow the play set hitter to move around the quick hitter's approach. The setter again uses a quicker release and allows the ball to be hit as it reaches its peak or slightly thereafter. The play set timing should remain fairly constant so the hitters will be able to time their approaches the same each time.

In advanced volleyball, *plays* are called that give the players their assignments as to how to cover the court, where to make the pass, the target and height of the set, the attacker, and possibly the direction of the spike.

The *height and placement of the set* in elite volleyball are determined by the play called. The placement may be to a front-court attacker or behind the three-meter line to a back-court spiker. In recreational volleyball, the set is usually sufficiently effective if it is two to three feet from the net and about 15 feet high. This gives the attacker sufficient time to make corrections in the approach and to make the hit.

Considerations for the setter at the more advanced levels are extensive. The setter is the quarterback of the team. It is up to the setter to understand the mood of the team during a match and to evaluate the performance of the attackers. Is one player having a "hot" day? If so, perhaps he or she should receive far more of the sets. By so doing, the setter may instigate a hot streak that may win the game.

The setter must be aware of the opponent's defense. How are the defenders defensing a crossing pattern by the attackers?

The setter must also think defensively. When the ball is in the opponent's court, the setter must play the assigned defensive responsibility first, then move to the setting position. Once you have moved to the setting position, let your teammates know that you are there. Call out "I'll set" or "I'm up."

Once the set is made, get into your defensive area of responsibility. And as the transition from defense to offense occurs, the setter is responsible for the second contact. If the setter is not able to make the second contact, it is essential to call the name of the player who should make the set.

Drills

Beginner

1. Assume the setting position and play with an imaginary ball. Flex your knees to get down to imaginary low balls. Check the position of your arms and hands. Are you holding your arms and hands in the proper position? Are you looking up through the space between your thumbs and fingers for the imaginary ball?

Incorrect foot position

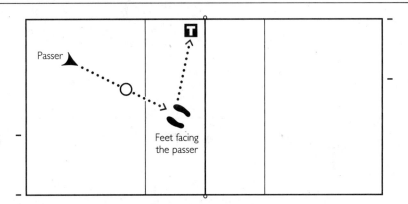

Correct foot position

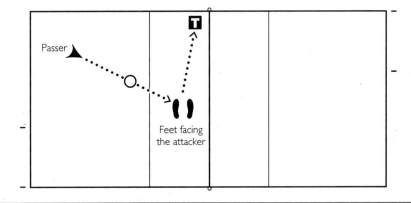

Off pass diagram:
Past and beyond

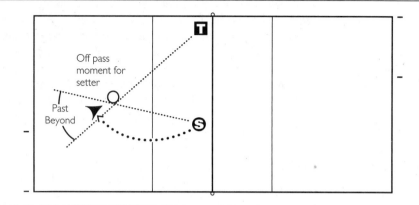

Play set

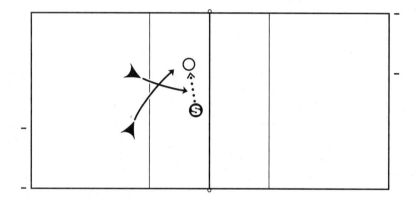

2. Hit the ball against the wall or to a partner. This can be done sitting, kneeling, squatting, and standing. In order to get used to setting a low ball, you can allow the ball to bounce from the floor, then set. Check on your elbow and hand position. When doing the drill standing, make certain that you move your feet properly and that your legs work with your upper body during the setting action.

3. With partners, set the ball, turn 360 degrees to the right, set the ball again, then turn 360 degrees to the left and set it once more. Spot the ball as quickly as possible and move your feet to the proper area as you prepare to make contact. Vary the distance between the partners and the height of the sets. Concentrate on the ball and beat the ball to the spot where it will be contacted.

Checklist for Progression in Learning Settings

Beginner-level skills

1. Overhand passing (setting) a tossed ball
2. Setting a passed ball

Intermediate skills

3. Setting "off" passes
4. Back setting
5. Underhand setting
6. Quick setting

Advanced skills

7. Running set
8. Jump set
9. Play set
10. Cross-court set
11. One-hand set
12. Using deception in setting to reduce the blockers' keys

Intermediate

4. With one partner standing on the attack line and the other on the back line, have the partners move along the lines while they set. The player on the back line will set diagonally, forcing the attack-line player to move to the spot. The attack-line player then sets straight ahead to the spot where the back-line player has moved. The back-line player sets straight ahead. The attack-line player sets diagonally to the attack-line player. The progression is hit straight twice, then hit diagonally once.

Saving ball out of top of net

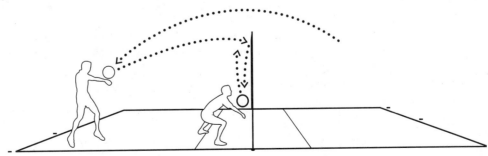

Saving ball out of bottom of net

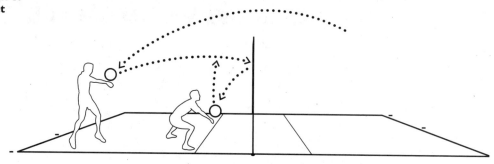

Endline setting drill

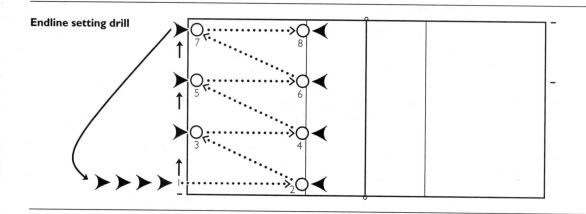

Advanced

5. Your partner or teacher stands in center court (zone 6). The setter (you) moves to the assigned area for the set (zone 3), then executes a front or back set to one of the two spikers positioned on the attack line.

6. The setter starts in left back position (zone 5), and the partner or teacher stands in right back position (zone 1).

7. *Triangle setting.* Passer to setter to target. The target can be a person or an object on the floor.

8. *Four-person with server tossing.* The server tosses over the net, the passer passes to the setter, and the setter sets to the target.

9. *Repetitive setting (setter pressure).* The coach or passer rapidly makes passes to setter, so that the passes are coming from different directions and at different heights in quick repetition.

10. *Team service.* Receiving for total setter-hitter continuity.

11. Perform the sets in game-related situations with the live passers and attackers.

Four-person pass set drill

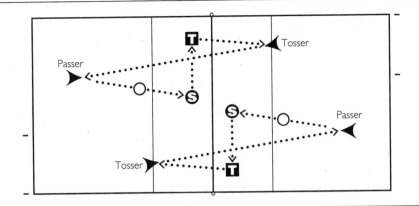

Setter release drill: Setter starts in the right back, goes to the net, sets either front or back, and then returns to the right back position.

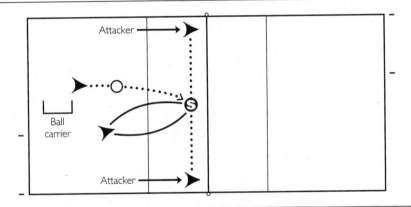

Setter left back release drill: Setter starts in the left back, goes to the net, sets either front or back, and then returns to the left back position.

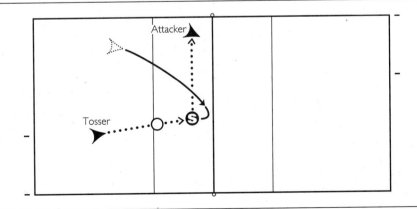

Triangle setting drill

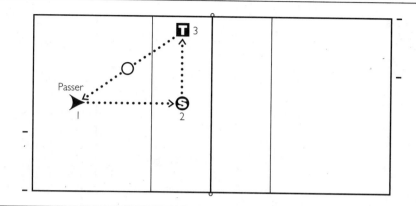

Summary

1. The set is a well-controlled overhand pass to an attacker.
2. The set should be made at the correct height and aimed to the exact spot for the attacker to make the kind of attack planned.
3. In correct setting, the setter must:
   a. Move under the ball quickly.
   b. Be able to generate sufficient power through a combination of leg and arm extension. (The arm extension is primary.)
   c. Control the ball with the pads of the fingers.
4. Sets can be made from a standing position to a position forward of or behind the setter, and can be made while running or jumping.
5. The setter is the quarterback of the volleyball team and must be aware of running the play system and controlling the game.

7

The Attack

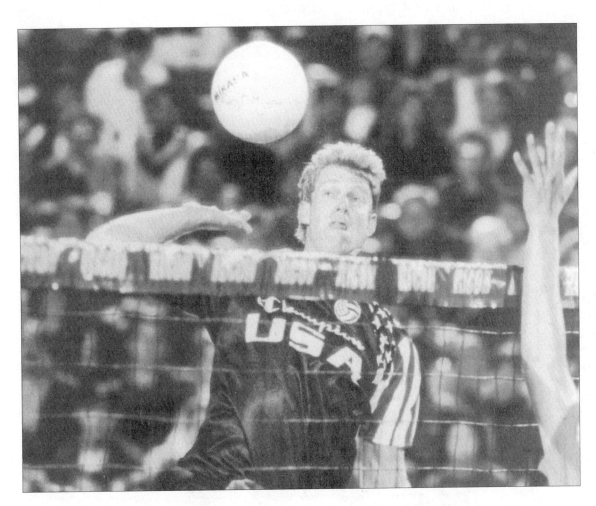

Outline

Т he attack is the last hit made by the offensive team. It is usually a hard spike, but may be a soft hit just over the blockers (called a "tip" or a "dink"), or a "roll" shot into an open area of the court.

Usually the attack is made on the third contact, but depending on the defensive court coverage or on a variation of offensive strategy, the attack might be on the second or even the first contact of the offensive team. The spike is the most exciting part of a volleyball game.

The Spike

The *spike* is the major offensive weapon of a volleyball team. It is made by the spiker jumping high and contacting the set ball at the maximum height attainable. The spike is then hit hard, usually with top spin, to direct the ball downward into the defenders' court.

The ability to control the body in the air while applying maximum power to the hit is essential to an effective attack. There are three elements of an effective spike: the approach, the jump, and the hit.

The *ready position* is similar in all sports. It allows the player to be able to move in any direction quickly. In the ready position, the player will start with the feet about shoulder width or slightly wider. The knees will be flexed. The torso will be bent forward at the waist. The weight will be on the balls of the feet. (Some players curl their toes to get the feeling of their weight being forward.) The arms will generally be bent and carried forward. The head will be up.

Once the potential spiker's receiving or defensive responsibilities have been met and the ball has been passed to the setter, the spiker will get to a position

Initial starting position

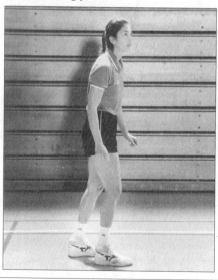

First step of the approach

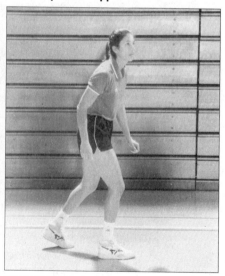

a. b. c.

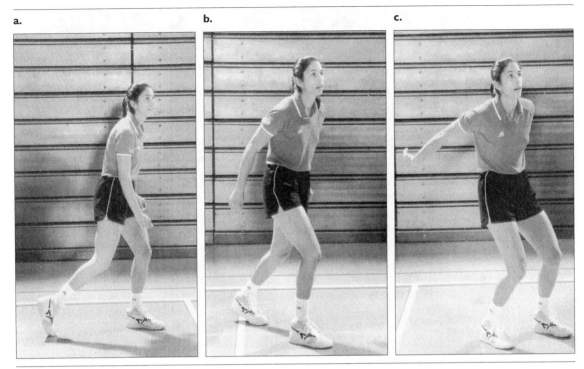

Approach:
a. Second step of the approach; b. Third step of the approach; c. Fast step (gather) of the approach with arms back

about 13 to 14 feet back from the net. The distance from the sideline will depend on the type of attack that has been planned. Beginners and intermediates are content just to hit a spike over the net, but advanced players are required to hit to a specific area, often with a special type of hit such as a sharp downward or a deep hit.

The *approach* can be four, three, or two steps. The number of steps depends on the height of the set and the position of the attacker. The standard four-step approach begins about four or more meters from the net. Starting that far away from the net has three advantages: it allows the spiker to generate horizontal speed that can be transferred into vertical lift on the jump; the hitter can adjust better to a set that is away from the net; and the spiker can adjust more effectively to a set that is made too far right or left of the spiker. (Beginning recreational players often stand at the net and expect to spike from there; but from this position they cannot adjust to a set, so the set would have to be perfect.)

The standard approach consists of four steps. The first step is a timing step. The second is a directional step toward the spot where the set will be spiked. The spiker will take the first step with the leg on the same side as the hitting arm (a right-handed hitter will take the first step with the right foot). The second step is a rather long one with the left foot. The next right-footed step will be short, as the horizontal drive of the first two steps is transmitted into vertical movement. The last step with the left foot stops the forward movement and

✓   *Checklist for the Spike*

1. Start about three to four meters from the net.
2. Your first step will be a timing step with your spiking-side leg. Your second step is a directional step toward the target.
3. Your last two steps finish with a gathering for the jump.
4. The ball should be hit 8 to 20 inches in front of the spiking arm.
5. The ball is hit with a reach and snap.
6. On landing, you (the spiker) must quickly prepare to play defense.

prepares for the jump. During the last two steps the knees are flexed and the "gathering" for the jump is completed.

The *jump* begins during the last two steps of the approach. The arms swing backward, then swing forward and up as the vertical jump is begun. The power for the jump comes from the front of the thigh (quadriceps muscles), the hips and rear of the thighs (gluteals and hamstrings), with a major thrust from the calf muscle (the gastrocnemius). The arms lead the body upward. The spiking arm is moved backward into the hitting position while the other arm points at

Jump:
a. Gather with double arm lift; b. Continuation of double arm lift and jump; c. Spiking arm drawn back in preparation for arm swing

a.

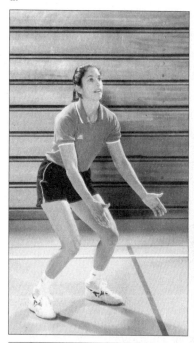

b.

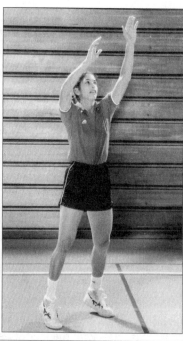

c.

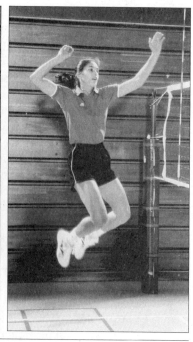

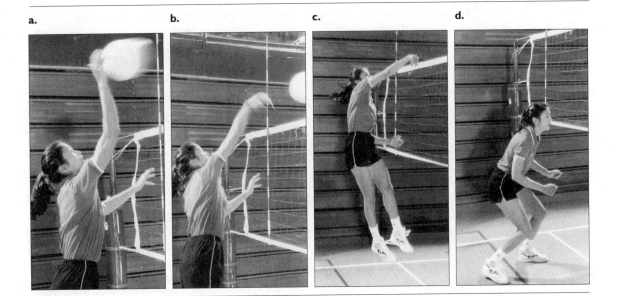

a.   b.   c.   d.

Jump:
a. Arm swing and contact; b. Wrist snap and follow-through; c. Spike follow-through; d. Post spike cushioned/landing

the ball to aid the concentration of the spiker. The back is arched to allow the abdominal muscles to stretch and begin the full body snap that delivers the power to the hit.

The abdominal muscles contract, bringing the hips around. Then the shoulders start their forceful movement forward. The legs straighten under the body with the contraction of the abdominals and the hip-flexing muscles. The non-hitting arm is pulled down as the spiking arm moves up and over the ball; these arm movements create a pinwheel effect.

Timing the hit takes practice. The approach should be delayed long enough so that the hitter is able to generate a great deal of speed and power, which will generate an explosive jump. This allows the hitter to reach the ball at the peak of the jump and contact the ball at the highest possible point.

A common error for spikers at all levels is to be over-anxious and to start the approach too early. This causes the player to run under the ball and lose power by having to slow down at the end of the approach.

The *hit* is akin to throwing a baseball but the ball is contacted out in front of the shoulder (8 to 20 inches, 20 to 50 centimeters). The top part of the palm of the hand, near the fingers, is the major contact point. The fingers then snap over the top of the ball and the hand rotates toward the target area of the court. (It is legal to hit with the fist, but it doesn't give any more power and there is much less control because not as much surface of the ball is contacted.) The wrist should be loose and allowed to snap freely, as if it were the end of a whip.

The *follow-through* will have the shoulders nearly perpendicular to the line of flight to the target. For a right-handed spiker in the right court doing a cross-court spike, the shoulders will be open toward the target. For a down-the-line

The hit

Side view of ideal arm and hand position

Back view of hand contact on ball

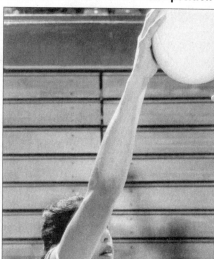
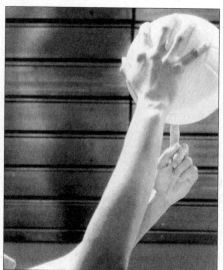

shot, the shoulders will not be rotated as far around. The force of the hit will have moved the body into a somewhat "piked" (bent forward at the hips) position. Then the legs will be brought back under the body while preparing to land. The eyes will stay on the ball to see if it has been killed.

The *landing* will be on the toes with the feet about shoulder-width apart. The attacker will then immediately assume the assigned defensive responsibility.

Keep the ball in front as the approach is made. The hitter should be able to see the ball and the block that is forming. With experience and practice, this becomes easier to do.

Other Types of Hits

The type of hit is determined by the hitter's personal arsenal of shots and the way the block has formed. For example, if the block is set inside, the hitter should be able to go down the line. If the middle blocker is late to close the block, the hitter should see this and hit the seam between the blockers. The hitter may also use a tip or an offspeed shot if an appropriate situation arises.

The *tip shot*, or *dink*, is a change-of-pace shot. It is a soft shot that may be made when an opening in the defense is spotted beyond the blockers or when the set is too poor to spike. At more advanced levels, it is generally made just over the head of the blockers to an undefended area, or, if there are no blockers, it may be made close to the net. The attacker must know where the defensive weakness is in order to use this skill effectively.

The tip is most effective when made after a fake. The spiker may prepare for

Tipping the ball

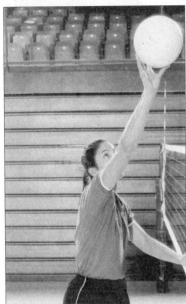

Hitting off the block

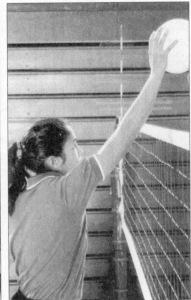

Wiping the ball off the block

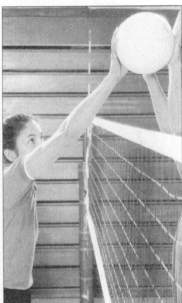

the hard hit, then, at the last second, softly touch the ball with the fingertips. The wrist and fingers must be stiff so that the ball leaves the fingers immediately and the player is less likely to be called for carrying the ball.

The *offspeed hit* is much the same as the tip, but the contact is made with the palm of the hand and the motion is the same as for the spike. However, instead of following through after the hit, the arm is slowed or stopped and the wrist snap places the ball over the block and into the open area of the court. This can be a very deceptive play.

The *wipeoff* is a shot used when the ball is set too tight to the net to allow the spiker to get it past the block. The approach must be quick and close to the net. The jump must be straight up to avoid going into the net. The ball is taken with the hand open and pushed into the blocker's arms. As the contact is made between the ball and the arms of the blocker, the offensive player turns the wrist outward and pushes the ball off the blockers' arms and out of bounds. Front-row setters can also use this shot on passes made close to the net in which the blockers may attack the set.

The *quick hit* is often the first option in a play system. A good quick hitter can contact the ball before the block is formed. A quick hitter must be fast enough to explode on the ball as the setter releases the set. Generally, the quick hitter will utilize a three-step approach. (Some coaches prefer four steps.) This allows for sufficient momentum to be built up but ensures that the attacker will be in the attack area at the moment that the low set should be hit. Players should be able to use the last two steps (the closing steps) from anywhere on the court. This allows them to step and gather for the jump with only minimal time expended. Unexpected or "off" plays and quick transition plays don't allow the hitter the time to make the preferred four-step approach.

Whatever the number of steps taken in the approach the hitter should make certain that the set will be hit far enough in front of the body so that the block can be seen forming. This allows the hitter to determine the type of spike or tip that will be most effective.

Quick hitters will also use an abbreviated arm swing. The backswing will not be extended much past the parallel point of the torso. By reducing the backswing, the armswing can be shortened and quickened.

To make the quick swing, the elbow should come up high and the body rotation should be lessened to enable a quicker snap of the arm. Once the arm is raised, the hitting action should follow immediately. The ball can be contacted as wide as the elbow of the spiking arm or as far inward as the midline of the body. The faster the arm action, the harder the hit. The ball should then be directed with the upper arm and the turn of the wrist.

For *playset hitting*, the second hitter delays, then breaks off the quick hitter for a set slightly higher than the quick hitter can reach. Since the set should also be off the net, the playset hitter will "long jump" more to the spot of the set and will explode into the ball.

By delaying and making a late break, the hitter can cause the block to jump with the quick hitter or be late in forming. This will allow the hitter more areas or seams into which to place the ball, as well as helping the hitter to be more explosive and hit the ball harder.

Starting position for back-row attack

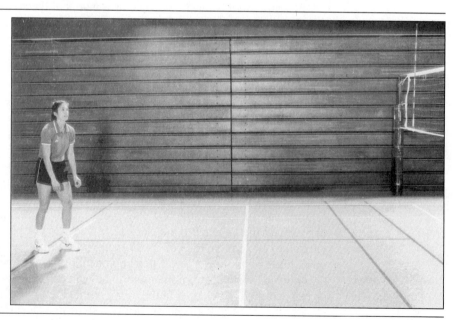

First step of approach for back-row attack

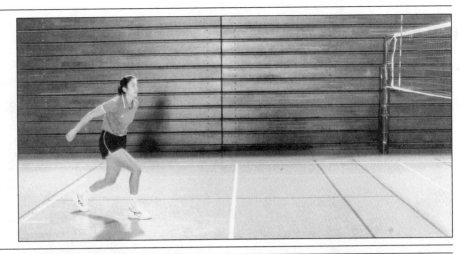

Second step of approach for back-row attack

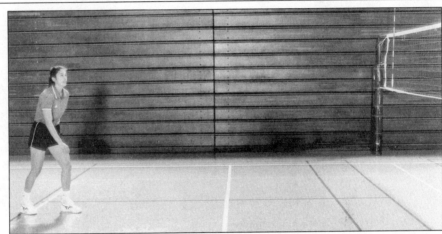

Gather with arms back

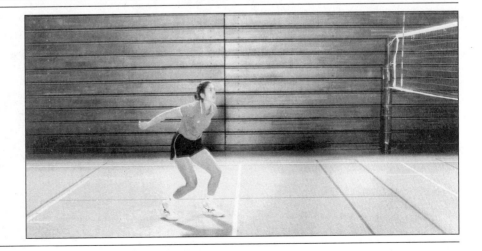

Double arm lift in preparation for long jump

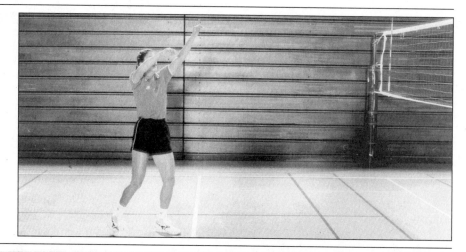

Long jump with arm in spiking position

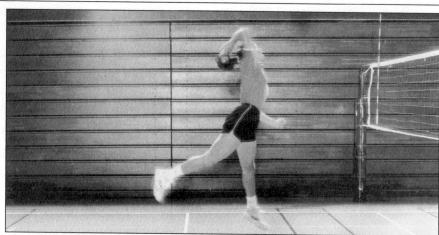

Arm moving just prior to contact

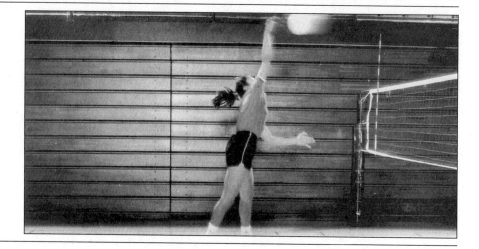

**Swing-hitting
movement**

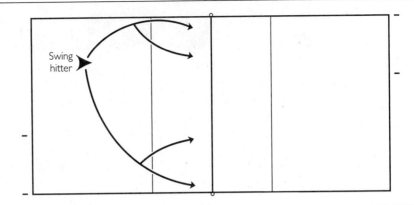

The *back-row attack* has been used more often in recent years to offset the larger and stronger blockers. The back-row attack allows the offense to incorporate virtually any hitter, whether in the front row or back row, into offense.

One of the major benefits of the back-row hit is the fact that, since the ball is contacted farther off the net, the attack angles are less acute and the ball becomes harder to block. A good hitter will develop both a cross-court and a down-the-line hit, enabling the hitter to attack a poorly formed or drifting block.

The approach will be from two or three meters behind the three-meter line, but instead of jumping straight up on the last steps, the hitter will long jump over the three-meter line. (As long as the attacker takes off from behind the line, the ball can be hit forward of the line.) The placement of the set will be determined by the spiker's jumping and hitting ability. The placement should permit the hitter to spike the ball when at the peak of the jump.

Swing hitting is a term brought into use in recent years to describe the activity of an attacker who has the ability to move (swing) from one area of the court to another to spike. This movement can confuse the blockers.

A swing-hitting player may be lined up in the left forecourt, then swing to the right forecourt to spike. This type of movement keeps the defense off balance and makes it difficult for them to commit their blockers by watching only the potential hitters who are near the set.

The *one-foot attack* has become an effective play to beat or move large blockers by creating quick movement laterally along the net. The player will move along the net and jump off of one foot to attempt to drive past where the blockers set up. Normally, right-handed hitters break to the right and left-handed hitters to the left.

The *lob* is a shot directed over the opposing players into an open area. It is used in the hope that it will force the defenders into the back court and bring about a poor pass. The lob is contacted from behind and below the ball.

Checklist of Common Errors in Spiking

1. Having the hand contact the underside of the ball rather than behind and on top of the ball.
2. Lifting with only one arm during the jump.
3. Hitting with a closed hand.
4. Overrunning the set so that the ball is behind, rather than in front of, the hitter.
5. Not having the nonspiking shoulder facing the net.
6. Keeping the elbow too low

Drills

1. *Outside-in hitting.* The attacker starts three meters from the net and from outside the sideline.

Outside-in hitting

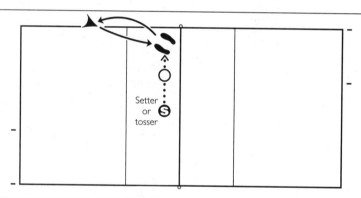

2. *Four-way step close.* A two-step drill in which the attacker goes forward, right, left, and back, hitting a tossed ball after each movement.

Four-way step close:
Player uses only
two steps (step close)
to spike balls that
are tossed one at a
time to the four
areas shown

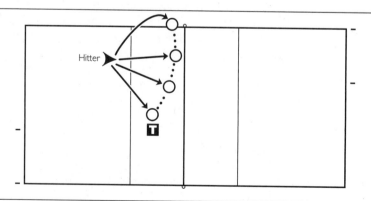

3. *Multiple-area deep hitting.* The attacker hits the ball to designated areas of the court.

Court placement

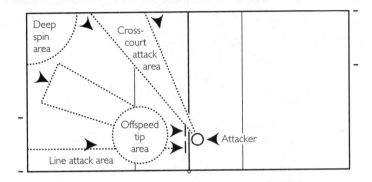

4. *Power and vision.* The teacher stands on a box on one side of the net and moves his or her arms right or left in a blocking motion. The attacker, who is on the other side of the net, hits a set or tossed ball opposite the direction in which the teacher moves his or her arms.

Multiple-area deep hitting

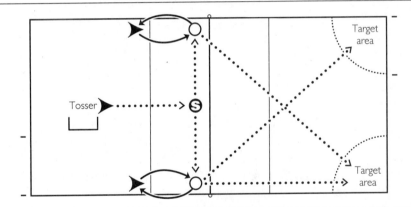

Power and vision: Attacker tries to hit the ball away from the blocker

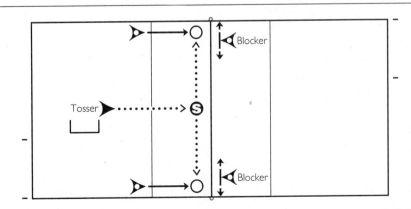

Checklist for Progression

Beginner

1. Jump and swing
2. Approach
3. Arm lift and arm snap

Intermediate

4. Tip shot
5. Offspeed hit
6. Lob

Advanced

7. Wipeoff
8. Quick hit
9. Playset hit
10. Back-row attack
11. Swing hitting
12. One-foot attack

Summary

1. The attack is the last hit made by the offensive team.
2. Generally, the most effective hit is a spike.
3. The spiker generally starts the approach from three to four meters back from the net.
4. There are several types of spikes, such as the play set hit, the quick hit, and the back-row attack.
5. Other types of attack hits are the: tip shot or dink, the offspeed, the wipeoff, and the lob.

8 *Blocking*

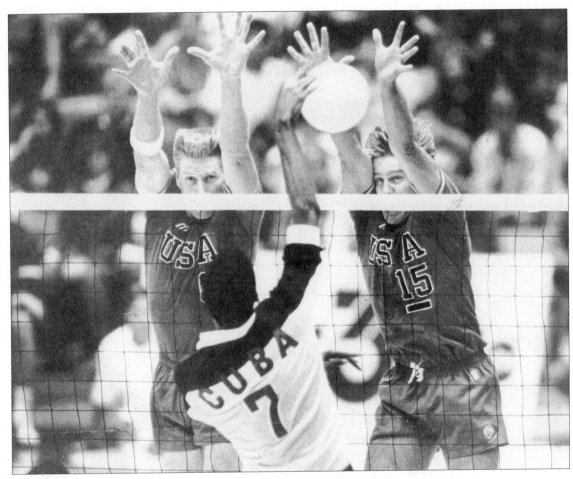

Outline

Blocking is a key defensive tactic in volleyball. It is the first line of defense against an attack. Properly executed, it eliminates or reduces the effectiveness of the attack. However, at the very beginning level it is not too important because there are not many spikes to block. Also, unless a player can reach over the net, he or she should not block. Such a player will be more effective in court coverage than by jumping up next to the net.

The most important concept to remember when blocking is that the ball must be intercepted on the opponent's side of the net. Because of this requirement, blocking is a very complex skill that must be constantly practiced—just as with any other skill.

Blocking is one of the most difficult skills to learn because it is difficult to break it up into its many parts and practice each part individually. The best way to learn to block is to execute the entire movement at 100 percent effort—physically and mentally.

The block can be made by one, two, or three players. The most common blocks are the two- and three-person blocks.

For years the teaching and coaching emphasis has been on all aspects of offense, individual defense, and ball control, while blocking techniques and tactics have been overlooked. Most of the available information on blocking is concerned only with technique. This chapter will address both the techniques and tactics of blocking.

The *starting position* for a block is at arm's length from the net. The knees will be slightly flexed and the hands at head height or higher in a ready position. (The better the pass, the higher the hands.) The eyes watch the ball, the setter, and the potential hitters in order to anticipate where the spike is likely to occur.

Initial starting position

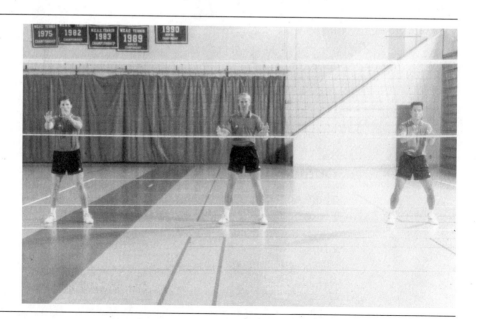

Side view of starting posture showing measure

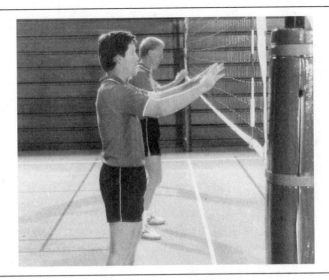

The two outside blockers are within three steps from their nearest sidelines and are at least one yard from the middle blocker. This enables the middle blocker on an outside set to take a big step and not interfere with the outside blocker.

The Eye Contact Sequence

The blockers watch the passed ball to the apex of its flight. If the ball is passed over the net, the blocker should hit it hard. If the pass is good, the blocker should prepare to block by reading the setter and the setter's release. It is desirable for the blockers to observe the attacker out of their peripheral vision, but

Eye contact sequence starts by watching setter

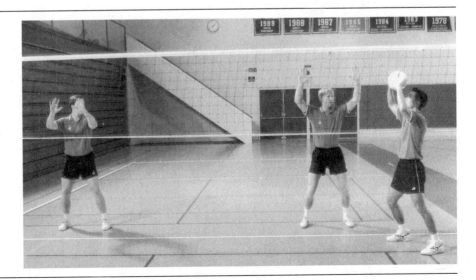

Blocker takes second step and watches hitter

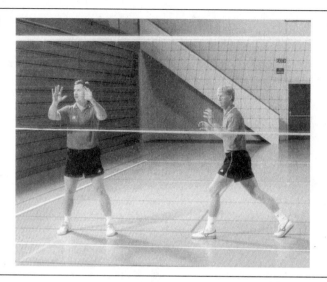

their visual focus should be on the setter and the setter's release. All sets can be judged by the initial speed of the ball. The eye contact sequence can be reduced to "ball-setter, ball-hitter."

Reading the setter is a way to anticipate the height and direction of the set. It allows the blocker to move quickly to the area of the attack.

- A setter with low hand positioning will often set low and to the outside.
- A shoulder dropped toward the net may tip off a short set to the middle.
- A setter moving farther under the ball may be tipping off a back set.
- A full extension of the knees is likely to indicate a high set.
- The direction of the follow-through indicates the direction of the set.

Blocker watches hitter and penetrates the net

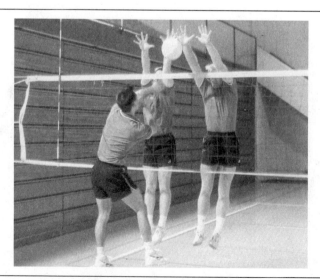

Reading the attacker is the next part of the eye contact sequence. Once the blocker identifies where the set is going, the blocker's focus changes from the ball to the attacker. The longer the blocker looks at the attacker, the more the blocker is able to observe. The blocker's reaction is slowed if the look is only momentary. The blocker should "read up" the hitter by identifying the attacker's point of origin and the attacker's line of approach, and culminate with a visual fix on the attacker's hitting shoulder and hitting arm. The final point of focus is watching the hitter contacting the ball. The blocker's eyes must remain open.

Footwork

There are two types of footwork patterns in blocking: the shuffle and the crossover. The shuffle is used to cover short distances of up to one or two yards. The crossover is used to cover more ground in setting up for a block. Whichever pattern is used, the feet must move into the proper position because the block is set with the feet, then the ball is blocked with the hands.

Shuffle step—stuffing ball to floor

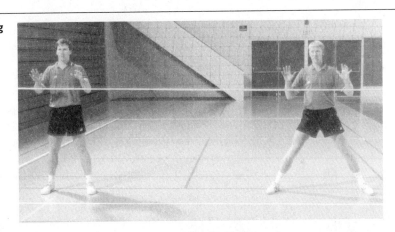

Feet together (gather)

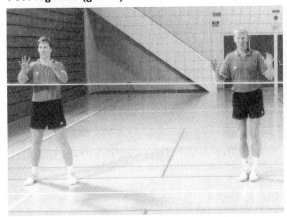

Second shuffle

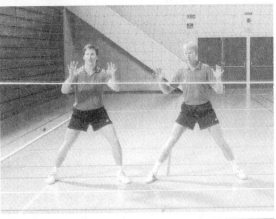

Gather for blocking jump

Blocking jump

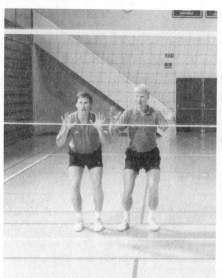

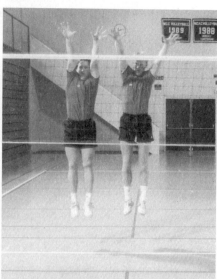

The *shuffle* is similar to the basketball defensive slide action, so it is easily learned by those who have played basketball. In the shuffle the leg nearest the target area is moved first; the trailing leg is then closed. The shuffle may be a series of two-step (step and close) movements. If these two steps get the blocker to the point of attack, the blocker prepares to jump as the trailing leg closes to the lead leg.

The *crossover* starts with a long lead step (the leg nearest the target), then the trailing leg crosses over in front of the leading leg—gaining the required distance. Then the lead leg closes and the blocker prepares to jump. This is normally a three-step movement, but it can be a five-step movement if the target area is a long way from the blocker. The crossover is similar to turning and running to the point of attack.

The problem with the crossover is that when the blocker finally arrives at the place where the block will occur, he or she must reorient to the net. This is done by facing the net, placing the shoulders square to the net, and positioning oneself the proper distance away from it—about arm's length. The blocker should always bend at the knees, not at the waist.

The jump of the blocker occurs just after the attacker jumps. The blocker will jump as high as possible while moving the arms over and across the net. The movement is not "jump up then put your arms over the net." The proper movement is "jump up while simultaneously sliding your arms across the net." This "seals" the net by not allowing space between the arms and the net in which the ball can go under the blocker's arms.

Checklist for Blocking

1. Be in the ready position at arm's distance from the net.
2. Watch the ball as it is set.
3. Move to where the ball will be hit.
4. Watch the hitter as you move and jump.
5. Jump just after the hitter jumps.
6. Extend your arms over the net (penetrate and seal) as you jump.
7. Reach as far into your opponent's court as possible. The ball must be intercepted on the opponent's side of the net.
8. Watch the hitter's arm and shoulder as the ball is contacted.
9. Read—setter to hitter.

Armwork

Net penetration (extending the arms over the net) is essential for making an effective block. The blockers must penetrate the opponents' air space as deeply as possible without touching the net. The angle of the arms should direct a blocked ball downward toward the center of the opponent's court.

The blockers should be able to perceive the backs of their hands in their peripheral vision field as they watch the attacker strike the ball. This will help to ensure that the hands are over the net, rather than merely above the net. It

Back view of blocking form

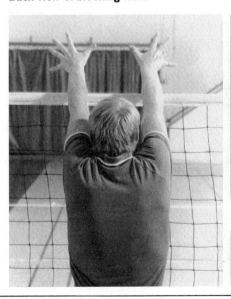

Side view of net penetration

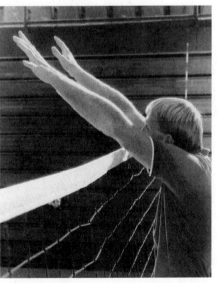

Checklist of Common Errors in Blocking

1. Attempting to block when you are unable to reach over the top of the net.
2. Staying with the set ball too long rather than reading the attacker.
3. Having your body too close to the net, resulting in a netting error and no penetration.
4. Having your arms straight up in the air.
5. Waving your arms excessively.

also helps the blocker to put his or her hands either on the ball or in the area in which the ball may travel.

The *arm position* will be fully extended with the fingers spread, the thumbs nearly touching, and the little fingers turned outward as far as possible. The fingers should be spread to take up as much area as possible.

Good blockers block balls with their hands, not their arms. The outside blocker should cover the attacker's hitting arm to take away the straight spike. The middle blocker takes away the attacker's cross-court shot.

As soon as the spike has occurred or the block has been made, the arms are quickly brought back to the blocker's side of the net. The body straightens out as it prepares to land.

Blocking Tactics

Blocking systems can be categorized as either the read or the commit-stack. In the read system, all blockers read the setter and then react to the set. The blocker's weight distribution is neutral and the blocker does not move until the direction of the set is read.

Stack blocking left-side set

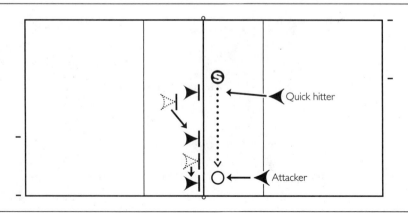

**Read blocking
for a right-side
attacker**

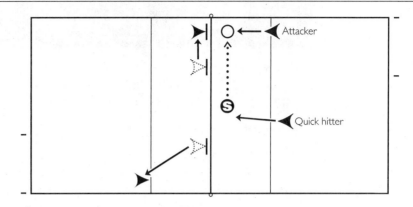

**Stack blocking
left-side set**

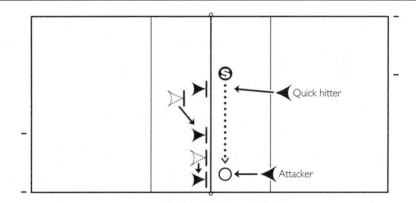

In the *commit-stack* scheme the blockers are aligned one behind the other in a stack. The first blocker takes out the quick hitter and tries to block the quick attack if it should come. This is the sole responsibility of the first blocker.

The stack blocker aligns behind the commit blocker then breaks right or left depending on the set or the movement of the playset hitter. The stack blocker can read the setter or follow a designated hitter.

**Stack blocking
right-side set**

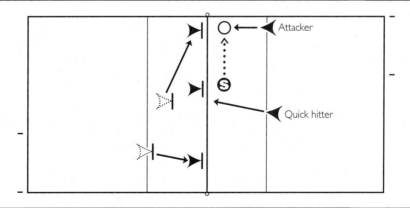

> ✓   *Checklist for Progression*
>
> **Beginners**
>
> 1. Eye contact
> 2. Block jump
>
> **Intermediate**
>
> 3. Footwork pattern
> 4. Arm movement
>
> **Advanced**
>
> 5. Read, commit/stack techniques
> 6. Read the attacker's approach and armswing

Drills

1. *Blocking while standing.* This is done by lowering the net to about four and one-half to five feet or by having the players stand on a table. An attacker on the opposite side of the net tosses the ball just above the net on his or her side of the net. The blocker stuffs the ball down to the floor while remaining standing. Each player should stuff about ten balls.

2. *Offspeed hit to target.* This is performed with the same lowered net or table. A hitter hits an offspeed (slowed up) spike to a predetermined spot. The blocker, knowing the direction of the hit, stuffs the ball to the floor.

3. *Penetrate and return.* This is learned by using the same props as above (low net or table). One player tosses the ball easily, just above the net. The blocker reaches over the net, catches the ball, and returns the arms quickly to his or her side of the net.

4. *Hand position.* This is reinforced by using the same low net or two tables (one for the teacher/coach and one for the two blockers). The teacher hits into the block while watching the hand position of the blockers. The outside blocker must have the hand turned in to stop the "wipeoff" shot.

5. *4-1-5 offense.* Three blockers work against three hitters using a 4-1-5 offense only. (4-1-5 offense: A ball is set to zone 4, a 51 set, or a 95 set. See Chapter 10, Systems of Team Attack, for the numbering system.)

6. *Reading and reacting.* Three blockers block against any offense. Emphasize reading the setter and reacting to the set.

7. *Block and recover.* This is drilled by having the teacher, who is standing on a table, use two balls. One ball is hit into the block then the second ball is tossed near the net to force the blockers to recover from the block and play the ball, which is now on their side of the net.

8. *Joust, overpass, and transition.* In this advanced drill, each team has three blockers starting at the net. One person tosses balls from alternating sides of the net. There are three options:

   a. The ball can be tossed above the net for the opponents to joust against one another.

   b. The ball can be tossed to the opposite side of the net for an attacker to hit as if in an overpass situation with the opponent blocking.

   c. The ball can be tossed to one of the diggers on either side while the front row drops off in transition.

   Each ball is played out to its completion. The game is rally-scored to 15 points. You can change the front row to back at eight points to keep the match-ups changing.

Summary

1. The block is one of the most difficult skills to master in volleyball.
2. The blocker should constantly measure the distance to the net.
3. The blocker must see the ball as it is passed and set, then move toward the area of the attack.
4. The blocker jumps while extending the arms over the net to seal and to penetrate the opponent's area.
5. The blocker must watch the attacker contact the ball.
6. The ball should be blocked to the center of the court if possible.
7. There are two blocking schemes, the read and the commit-stack systems.

9 *Individual Defense*

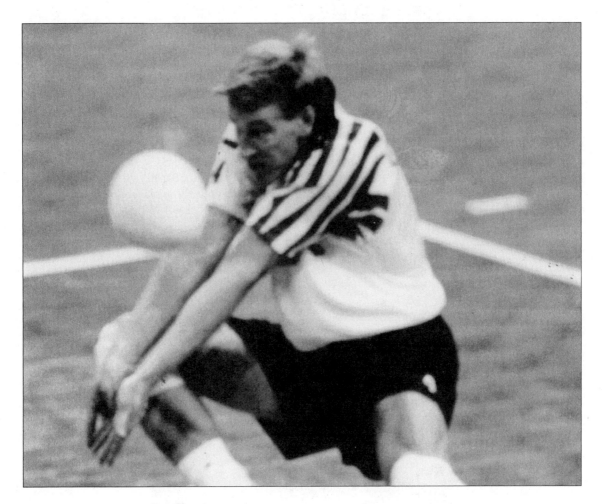

Outline

Defense is as much an attitude as it is a learned skill. Players should obviously use good positioning and skills, but they must also have an attitude that makes them eager to pursue balls that do not go directly to them.

Executing an Effective Defense

The *skill part of defense* is a combination of balance and the ability to rebound the ball up on the player's side of the court with control. The pass must be high enough for the setter to handle it effectively and it must be targeted so that the setter can play the ball from the desired area.

Positioning is extremely important prior to the opponent's attack. The defensive positioning on the court is determined by the type of team defense being used. (This subject will be discussed more fully in Chapter 11, Team Defense.)

The *ready position* begins with the feet about shoulder-width apart and with the weight forward and on the toes. A slightly staggered stance with the right foot forward is the preferred method because it standardizes the fundamental. If the right foot is always forward on every contact, the player doesn't have to learn the different weight shift that would be necessary if the left foot were sometimes forward.

Some teachers prefer that the outside foot be forward, because this might help the player to pass back into the court. This allows for "on help" (meaning

Individual defense ready position

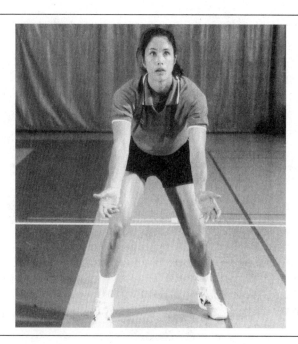

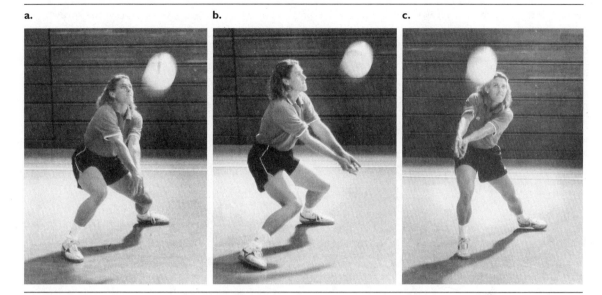

a.

b.

c.

Digging:
a. Posture for digging;
b. Posture for digging a hard drive spike;
c. Posture for digging a ball outside the midline of the body

that there is help on the inside of the court if a mistake is made on the pass).

The defensive player may be in a stationary position or may pre-hop just prior to the ball being contacted by the attacker. This is similar to the action of a tennis player preparing to receive a serve. The stationary position is recommended because the pre-hop often takes the weight from the toes and shifts it to the heels—the least desired weight distribution.

The arms extend in front and away from the body. They should be in the passing position prior to the contact of the ball. The keys to digging with con-

Posture for digging up using the "J" stroke

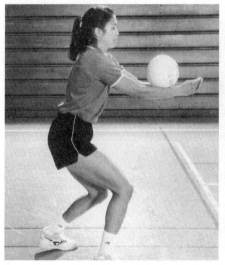

Front view of "J" stroke posture

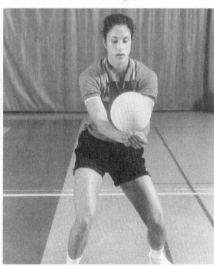

Striding into the defensive sprawl　　**Stride and extension prior to contact**　**Digging the ball with the sprawl**

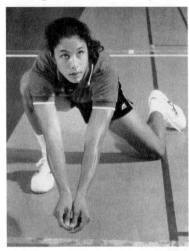
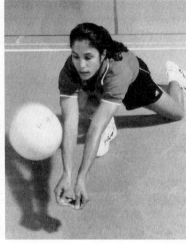
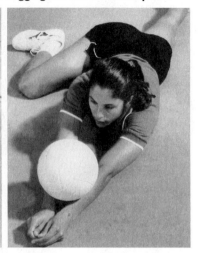

trol are to keep the rebound angle of the arms always pointing up and to move the feet so that the ball can be played in the midline of the body. This is called the "stride" or "lunge."

This striding movement should be used to get low and under the ball. The foot closest to the ball leads, so the balance and support remains inside the midline of the body. The greater the stride, the better the player's range becomes. The ball should be contacted low and on the forearms. The wrists snap up to scoop or "J" the ball up with backspin. On harder-hit balls, the player may need to take speed off the ball by cushioning it so that it doesn't

Posture prior to striding to the ball　**Striding to the ball with first step**　**Striding to the ball with second step**

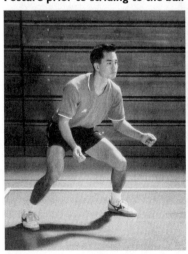
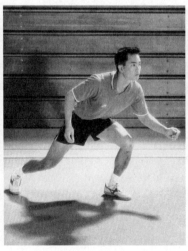
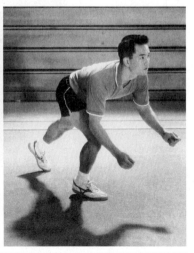

Playing the ball up with a dive

Post dive catch and slide

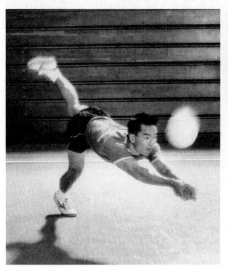 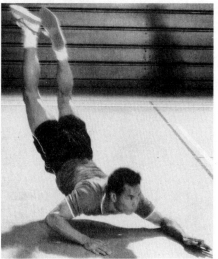

rebound back over the net. This action is gained by moving the arms slightly back toward the body upon contact with the ball.

The *sprawl* is one of the techniques used to increase the range of one's play. It is used when the ball is outside the range of the player's stride. After extending to the full reach of the stride, the player continues to move to the ball by extending the body parallel with the floor. The ball is played outside the midline of the body. The arms are thrust forward and kept parallel to the floor. The ball is scooped just before contacting the floor, and the player finishes the play by laying out flat on the floor.

The *dive* is a further extension of the sprawl. In the dive, the player moves toward the ball, then dives along the floor. This move is used when a player has generated momentum by running after the ball; it is the recovery move used after the ball has been played.

As in all defensive save techniques, the ball should be played as close to the floor as possible. Since the ball is close to the floor, the body will also be low. The play can be made with one hand, but two hands are preferable.

After the ball has been played, the hands are extended to the ground and the weight of the body supported to cushion the landing. As the chest and abdomen get close to the ground, the back is arched and the feet kicked up to avoid dragging the knees and toes. The head is held up to keep the chin from contacting the floor, and the hands are pushed back along the sides of the body to gradually dissipate the momentum of the body weight landing on the floor.

If executed properly, the dive recovery will allow the player to make a good controlled play and then get to the floor with no injury. The recovery should be trained without the ball to ensure proper technique. Once the technique is perfected, the ball can be introduced and the whole process can be practiced.

Checklist for the Save Technique

1. Start in the ready position.
2. Have your outside foot forward.
3. Keep your arms in front of your body and ready to handle the hit.
4. Move your feet so that the ball can be played in the midline of your body.
5. Keep the rebound angle of your arms pointing upward—"Dig up, not out."
6. Contact the ball low and snap your wrists up to give the ball backspin.
7. Use an appropriate recovery technique.

The *roll* is another save technique. It is used when the ball is beyond the reach of a stride or a sprawl. In the roll the player will once again try to play the ball from the lowest position possible. The stride is made and the body weight extended over the lead leg. The ball is contacted with either one or two hands and the wrist is snapped up to control the ball and give it backspin.

Once the ball has been played, the recovery process is started by the knee of the lead leg turning back toward the body so that the torso is turned to expose the player's back rather than his or her side. From this position there are a couple of ways to continue the recovery. In the log roll, the player simply rolls across the back laterally. In the somersault roll, the player rolls diagonally across the back and over the opposite shoulder—a back shoulder roll. If performed correctly, this momentum allows the player to roll back to the ready position.

Extending to play the ball	**Post contact "log roll"**	**Completion of the "log roll"**
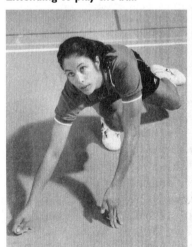	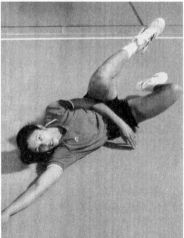	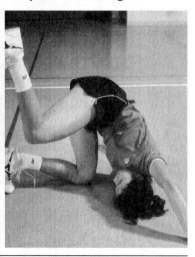

Checklist of Common Errors in Defensive Technique

1. Moving while the ball is being attacked.
2. Failure to watch and block the hitter.
3. Not pursuing the ball.
4. Digging the ball back over the net instead of to a setter.

In any technique the primary consideration is to make the play on the ball first, then make the recovery. Of course, even the best form on the dive or roll is useless unless the ball is properly hit and controlled.

Drills

1. *Two-table multiple contact digging.* Two tables are set up on one side of the net. One person stands on each table and tosses balls at the single digger on the other side of the net.

2. *2/3/4 person pass-set-hit.* The teacher or coach stands on a table and tosses a ball to a passer, who starts the pass-set-hit sequence.

3. *High-set ball defense.* The ball is set high to a hitter. The block forms and the nonblockers set up in their defensive alignment.

4. *Direct-set hitting drill.* The setter sets the hitter (no pass), and a block forms quickly.

5. *Advanced hitter coverage.* Two people with several balls are needed for this drill. The drill is run on one side of the net with no opponent. Person #1 puts the first ball into play to one of the defensive players or the hitter. The ball is dug and the setter sets to the hitter in the left-front position. The diggers and setter follow the ball to the hitter and move into their hitter coverage positions. Person #2 waits until the hitter makes contact with the ball and then tosses another ball to the coverage players. The ball is played up, set, and attacked again in transition. As the players become more proficient at their positions and coverage skills, additional balls from person #2 can be added. To increase the difficulty of the drill, person #2 can be put on a box or jump and throw the ball down to the hitter coverage group; this simulates balls that are blocked back with velocity.

6. *Advanced multiple digging.* Three hitters are on boxes. The hitter in the quick position starts the drill by hitting to the digger. After making that play, the digger move to make a play coming from the cross-court hitter. Then the digger drops back deep down the line to make a final play on the line hitter. With less skilled players, the digger must touch all three balls to

---

✓   *Checklist for Progression*

Beginner

1. Basic position
2. Digging ball up with two arms

Intermediate

3. Sprawl
4. Ball pursuit

Advanced

5. Dive
6. Roll

---

score a point. As the skill improves, the digger must *get* all three balls up to score a point. Finally, at the higher levels, the ball must be dug to a specific area to score. Begin the drill with the hitters giving the diggers plenty of time to get to the correct digging position on the court. The teacher or coach should focus on making sure the diggers are consistently getting into the correct position and using proper technique. As the diggers learn the correct movements and positions, decrease the amount of time they have to get to the spot and make the dig. Then add in tips and offspeed shots so the players learn how to react to something other than just hard-hit balls. To increase the difficulty and make the drill more game-like, add a blocker and have the player dig around that blocker. Have the hitter occassionally hit the ball off the blockers hand to get the digger to react to a ball that has been touched by the block.

Summary

1. Defensive play is as much an attitude as it is a series of skills.
2. The first concern is to position oneself properly to be able to perform the assigned responsibility for the team.
3. Be in the ready position before the ball is hit by the opponents.
4. Hit the ball as close as possible to the floor.
5. Use the stride, sprawl, dive, or roll techniques to reach the ball and recover from the save.

10 *Systems of Team Attack*

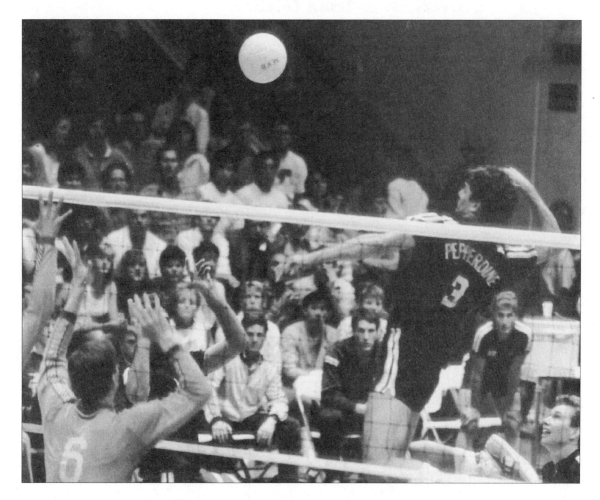

Outline

Every team has a basic system with which it works. The system is determined by the number of hitters and setters employed. Within the system, various formations are employed to receive the serve, attack the set ball, and cover the attacked ball.

Overview of Team Offense

Serve reception is extremely important in team offense, because without controlling the serve the team cannot attack effectively and gain the serve. When you are getting ready to receive, don't look at the server—concentrate on the ball.

Team offense begins with the service reception. While receiving service, the rule is that there cannot be an overlap between adjacent players (refer to Chapter 3). When a serve is hit, the front-row players on the receiving team must not duck under a ball if they are not going to pass it. Instead, players should "open up" by moving sideways. This will open a passing lane for the back-row passer.

Court formation with no illegal overlaps

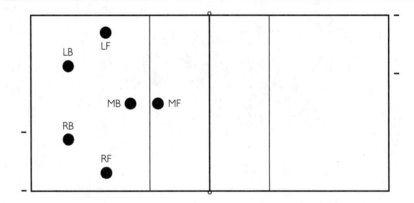

Court formation with illegal overlaps: Middle back must be behind middle front

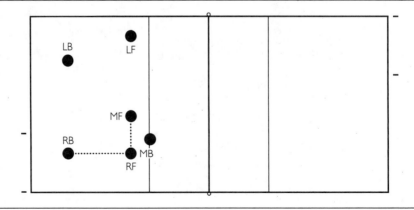

To *develop a team offensive system*, the team players' strengths and weaknesses must be identified. Once this is done, training should maximize the strengths and hide the weaknesses—so effective teams will use varying theories and strategies.

Common errors in developing an offense are:

- Trying to play a system beyond the team's skill level; never try to execute tactically what you are not capable of executing technically
- Failure to properly evaluate the players' strengths and weaknesses
- Not utilizing the potential of the players because of the limitations of the system being played
- A lack of specialization of skills for each playing position
- Improper use of the players in the starting lineup

Attack options include getting one or more spikers in a position from which they can successfully attack the ball. At the beginning level, there will generally be just one spiker on each side of the setter. At the intermediate level, a team may employ a single crossing pattern in which a quick hitter and a play set hitter cross, with either of them attacking the ball. (The setter will determine

Split hitters

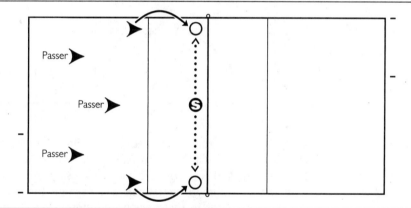

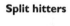**X-crossing pattern**

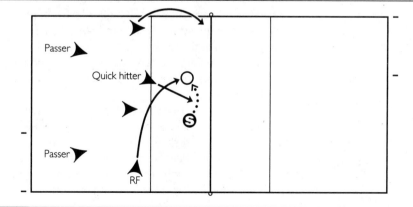

Multiple-crossing patterns

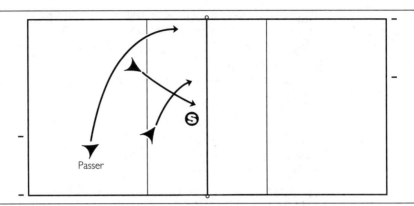

Passer

Advanced patterns

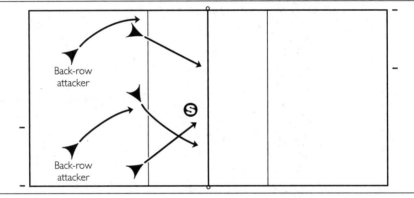

Back-row attacker

Back-row attacker

which player will receive the set.) At the elite level, there are usually multiple crossing patterns with as many as five possible attackers attacking—three from the front row and two from the back row—moving in the pattern at the same time. In this system the setter can predetermine the attack patterns and who will receive the set, or the specialized hitters can call out their attack patterns and the setter can then choose the best option to set.

Specialization is essential at the higher levels of play. The teacher or coach should determine the strengths of each player, then place them in an offensive scheme that permits those skills to best be utilized. The good passers must be put into positions where they can make most of the passes, the good setter should be doing most of the setting, and of course the good hitters should do most of the attacking.

For example, in a 5–1 offense (which will be discussed more fully later in the chapter) the player opposite the setter could be either a specialized passer or a specialized hitter-blocker who does not set in the normal serve-receive pattern.

As each player practices an area of specialization, he or she becomes far more proficient at that skill. This is a recent innovation in volleyball, but has long been the mode of operation for other sports such as baseball and football.

In developing an offense it is important to *practice in game-related situations*. While drills are important in developing skills, at the advanced levels scrimmaging should often be used early in the practice rather than late in the session. Additionally, a team should scrimmage often in practice. The major learning task for the day, whether it is techniques or team play, should be practiced early when the players' minds are fresh.

Offensive Systems

Beginner System

The *beginning offensive system* is a *6–6 system* of offense. The 6–6 means that all six players can be setters or attackers. Usually the player in the middle of the front court is the setter. After a rotation for the serve, that player becomes the right-side spiker and another player rotates into the middle setting position.

The *serve receiving formation* is the "W" formation. This formation uses three players about 14 to 15 feet from the net, and two deeper players in the seams

W formation

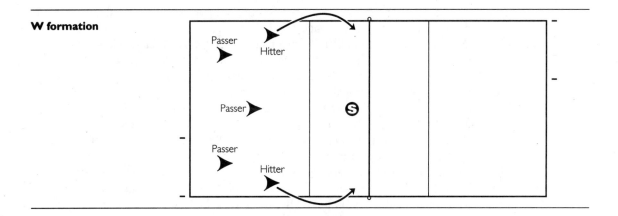

between them about 21 to 23 feet from the net. The setter aligns near the net closest to the center front (zone 3), being careful not to overlap side to side with the other front-row attackers. The pre-serve ready position will have each passer with the right foot forward, knees slightly bent, and arms in front of the body. By always having the right foot forward, only one motor skill is required no matter which zone is being served.

Whatever the serve receiving formation, the players should all be able to see the server and be ready to react to a serve in their respective areas. They should also know who is responsible for calling the lines (when a ball goes out of bounds). This is best done by having the two people deepest in the formation help the others. If the serve is going to the left-back player, the right-back player takes responsibility for making the call.

Hitter coverage

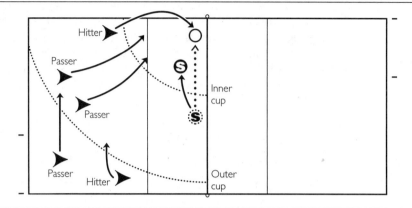

Both verbal and nonverbal communication among the passers is important, so a player may signal verbally with a call or may make a nonverbal signal by moving to or away from the serve.

In general, the front-row passers should not play a ball that is above waist height; they should let the back-row players take these. Players should also know who will take balls in the seams between them. An easy rule to remember is to have the player on the right of a seam take the balls served into the seam. But individual skills may require a different tactic—perhaps allowing the best passer to handle all balls in his or her area.

Hitter coverage is the action in which the attacking team members align to cover their court in the event that the spiked ball is blocked back into their court. In general, the receiver will pass the ball and then follow it to the net.

In hitter coverage, the eyes of the players should be on the arms of the blockers rather than on the flight of the ball from the spiker to the block. This is because it is much easier to focus on the ball as it comes off the block than as it leaves the hitter's hand before bouncing off the block. In any system of play, the hitter coverage formation should include an inner cup and an outer cup.

In the 6–6 system, the inner cup (three players closest to the attackers, forming a semicircle) will include the setter and the two back-court players nearest the attacker. The nonhitting attacker and the deepest back-court player play the outer cup. So if the attack is from the left forecourt (zone 4), the setter, the left back, and the center back form the inner cup and the right-front attacker and right-back player form the outer cup (players farthest from the attacker who form a secondary line in the seams between the members of the inner cup).

The advantage of the 6–6 system is that everyone gets to play every position and it is very simple. It gives beginners a chance to understand the game. The disadvantage at the higher levels of play is that the players generalize rather than specialize, so they are not able to adapt to their best positions. A short player who may have the potential to be a good setter gets to set only once in the six serve-receive rotations.

Intermediate System

The *intermediate system* is the *4–2 system* of offense. In the 4–2 system there are four attackers and two setters. In this system a setter will always be in the front row, so there will be only two attackers in the forecourt positions.

4–2 offense

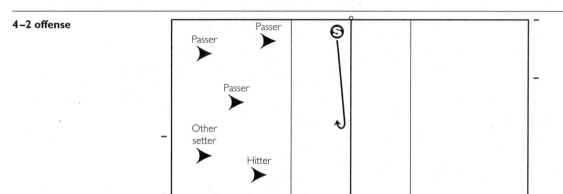

At the lower intermediate level the setter will generally be positioned in the middle of the front court—approximately ten feet from the right sideline. The attackers will be split on either side of the setter. If the setter is in a side zone, the attackers will align in the other two zones, to the inside of the setter.

Middle setter

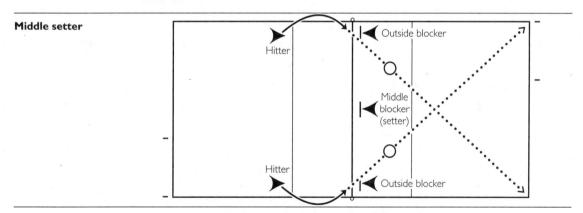

Advantages of the middle setter scheme include:

- The wider spiker has more area on the diagonal in which to hit the ball (42 feet across the court).
- The spiker has a better chance to intentionally hit off the block and out of bounds.

Advantages of the side court setter scheme include:

- It puts pressure on the middle blocker to first protect against an attack from the middle spiker and then move to the side if the set goes to the widest attacker.

- An attack from the center of the court is effective against some players.
- For teams that switch players into the block because they don't like their setters being involved in blocks at the center, this alignment of the offense reduces the possibility of such switches.

If the setter sets from the right-front zone (zone 2), the spiker who will play the left-side zone (zone 4) for two rotations [because he or she started in the left zone or switched with the setter who started in the center zone (zone 3), then moved to the left zone (zone 4)] is called the "on-hand" hitter. The spiker who stays twice on the right side [starting in the right zone (zone 2) or switching with the setter who started in the right zone] is called the "off-hand" hitter.

International 4–2

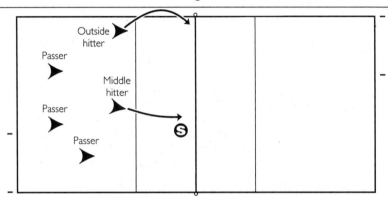

The *serve receiving formation* for the 4–2 is commonly the W formation (see the 6–6 formation described earlier). The 4–2 responsibilities are shown in the following diagram.

4–2 serve-receive responsibilities

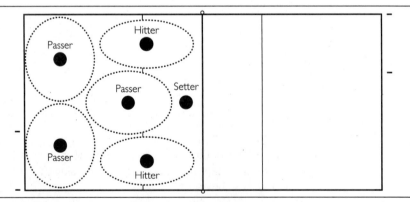

General advantages of the 4–2 offense include:

- There is less movement by the players, so theoretically errors are reduced.
- Less skilled players are more likely to be more efficient.
- It is a simple system, so tactics are usually easy to employ.
- It allows the small player to remain active in the game.

- It needs only two good hitters (because one can always be in the front line).
- The hitter coverage is strong.
- Passer accuracy is not as critical as in other schemes, since there is a larger target area (because the setter is always in the front row).
- It is a good system for an inexperienced coach.
- It is a good system for inexperienced players.

Disadvantages of the 4–2 offense include:

- It is difficult to deceive opponents with only two major attackers in the front row.
- There are only two attackers versus three blockers.
- Sets are received from two different setters, so the setters and hitters are not as familiar with one another.

In order to reduce these disadvantages, good teams make passes to the setter that are high enough to allow a setter to attack or set the ball. With a setter who can spike, the offense gains another option and the defenders have to defend against it. This is a prime time for the setter to use a jump set, because the blockers don't know whether to defend a spike by the setter or to defend against the remaining two hitters.

Hitter coverage in the 4–2 offense tends to be consistently strong because there are only two attackers to cover. The shift to the inner and outer cup responsibilities are the same as those explained for the 6–6 system.

When designing a *starting lineup* for this offense, the important consideration in placing the players is balancing their strengths and abilities. In respect to the six zones on the court, the best attacker should be positioned opposite the second-best attacker. The fourth-best hitter will be one zone clockwise of the best hitter. The third-best hitter will be opposite the fourth-best hitter. The best setter will be one zone clockwise of the fourth-best hitter. The second-best setter will be opposite the best setter. (See the diagram.) The intent is to place the best two hitters so that one will always be in the front row.

Typical starting position for a 4–2 offense

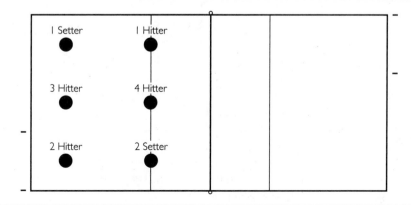

Checklist of Common Errors in Team Offense

1. Trying to play with a system beyond the team's skills
2. Failure to evaluate players' strengths and weaknesses
3. Not utilizing each player's potential because of the specific system's limitations
4. Not developing skill specialization for individual team members
5. Improper use of players in the starting lineup

The actual zones that the players take at the beginning of a game may depend on several factors. The coach may want the strongest server to be the first server, or perhaps it is more important to have the best hitter start in the left-front court. If, for example, the best server is also the best attacker, the coach will have to choose between these two initial starting positions. But in either case, the relationships described will remain intact. Another possibility for the starting rotation might be that the coach wants to receive serve and then rotate into the team's strongest blocking and defensive rotation.

Advanced Systems

Advanced systems of offensive volleyball are the 6–2 and 5–1. In the 6–2 system, all six players may be attackers but two are designated as setters. Currently at the elite level, a 5–1 is more commonly used; in this system there are five attackers and only one setter.

6–2 offense:
The two setters who are opposite each other come out of the back row to set. The three front row players all hit.

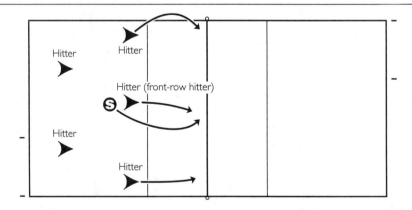

The *6–2 system* uses a back-row player as the setter so all three of the front-line players can be attackers. They can be employed in a variety of different alignments and patterns.

Advantages of the 6–2 offense include:

- There are more front-line attackers (three).
- The three attackers are better able to defeat three blockers.
- With three attackers it is tactically easier to attack the entire length of the net.
- There are multiple offensive possibilities.
- Players often prefer a three-hitter attack and so will work harder to perfect it.

Disadvantages of the 6–2 offense include:

- All six players must be adequate hitters.
- The serve must be received accurately.
- The setter must hit as well as set.
- The hitters must be able to adjust to the sets of two different players.
- Transitions are more difficult for inexperienced teams.
- It takes more time to perfect.
- Because the system is more difficult, players may blame the system for their own poor play.
- This system requires more jumping, more conditioning, and more practice time in order to be effective.

The *serve receiving formation* can be designed to receive with two, three, four, or five players. It is actually easier to receive serves with fewer people, because there is less chance of miscommunication between the potential receivers. The 1984 and 1988 men's Olympic gold medal teams, for example, employed a two-man serve receive formation. A "W" formation can be employed if five players are to be responsible for the serve reception; four players would play in a semicircle alignment; and two or three players receiving would be in a straight line (see diagrams).

Sample two-man serve receive

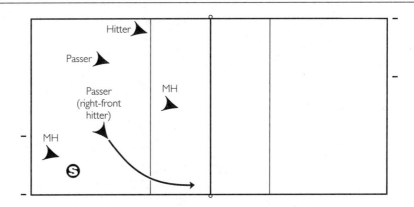

**Hitter coverage
on a quick hit**

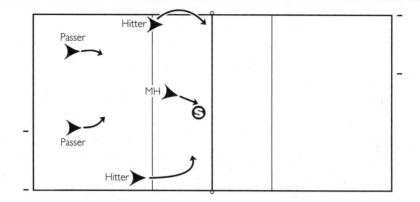

Hitter coverage for a middle attack would have the setter as the only player in the inner cup. This is because the setter is so close to the middle hitter and the blockers that it is easy to handle the ball blocked downward. The other four players form a close semicircle as the outer cup.

**Hitter coverage for
outside attack with
a quick hitter**

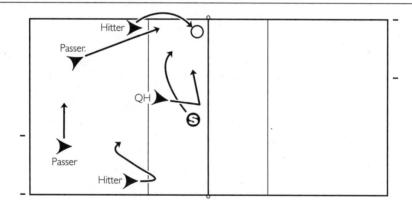

**Right side:
Hitter coverage**

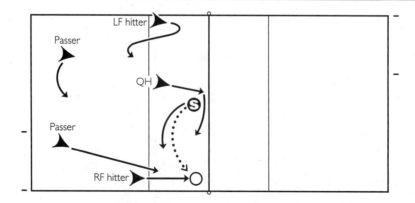

For an attack from the outside if the pass is good and the quick hitter jumps, the setter then moves to the area of the attack and becomes the primary member (the middle position) of the inner cup. The back-row player behind the hitter moves forward and becomes the deepest player in the inner cup. The quick hitter, after landing, moves along the net and becomes the inside member of the inner cup. The closer and lower the set is to the net, the tighter the inner cup will be. The center back and the offside attacker form the outer cup by positioning themselves in the seams of the inner cup but about ten feet behind.

If the pass is poor the setter can't make the quick set, so the quick hitter does not jump. The quick hitter then becomes the primary (middle) member of the inner cup and the setter takes the position by the net. In other words, on a poor pass the quick hitter and setter exchange responsibilities in the inner cup.

Sample 6–2 offense

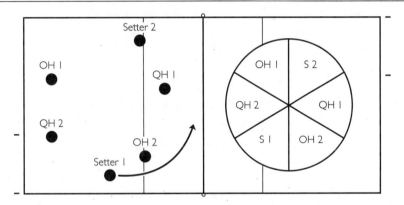

Designing a *starting lineup* for a 6–2 offense requires concerns similar to those mentioned for the 4–2. The 6–2 system generally has two specialized setters, two specialized quick hitters, and two specialized passer-outside hitters. As in the previously mentioned rotation, the setters will be opposite each other. In the rotation the quick hitters will lead the setters and the passer-outside hitters will follow the setters.

The *5–1 offense* uses one setter and five attackers. It is the most commonly used system in elite-level volleyball, from high school to the Olympics. With the setter in the back court the attack is like a 6–2, with three front-line hitters. When the setter is aligned in the front court it is like a 4–2, with only two primary hitters.

In this system, when the setter is in the front row, he or she must be able to jump set as well as tip or hit. With these skills, it is hoped that the setter can occupy one blocker.

The setter must be physically, technically, and emotionally fit. He or she must be intelligent enough to understand the complete game and intuitive enough to be able to direct the attack in a way most advantageous to the offense. The setter must know who is a "hot" hitter. It is also important to know where the matchups favor the offense so that the hitter chosen will have the best chance of defeating the block.

5–1 offense

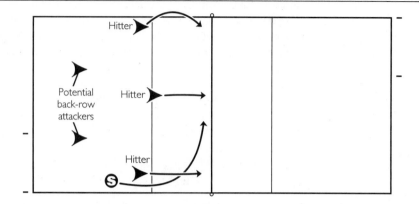

Advantages of the 5–1 offense include:

- Only one setter is in control all the time.
- Hitters need only learn to read (work with) one setter.
- Five hitter/blockers are always in the game.
- There are more potential combinations for attacking.

Disadvantages of the 5–1 offense include:

- A team must have one great setter.
- A team must have an accurate passing team to enable the setter to set, spike, or tip the ball when the setter is in the front row.
- There are three rotations where only two hitters are in the front line.

Formation for serve receiving is the same as in the 4–2 and 6–2 systems. Hitter coverage is the same as in the 4–2 and 6–2 systems, with the exception that all players must be aware of the setter's attempt to attack (tipped or spiked ball on the second contact).

5–1 offense:
Starting lineup

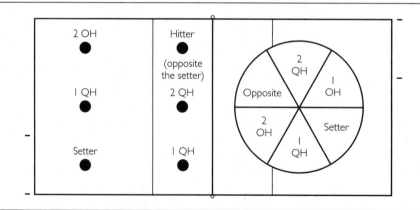

Designing a *starting lineup* for a 5–1 attack allows for more options by the offense than other systems do. The offense can be designed to take advantage of a number of specialized strengths of the team members. For example, the player opposite the setter could be a specialized right-side player, a specialized passer and left-side player, or a quick hitter/back-row attacker.

Swing offense

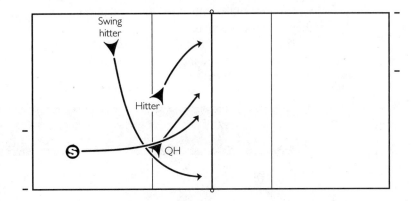

Swing offense

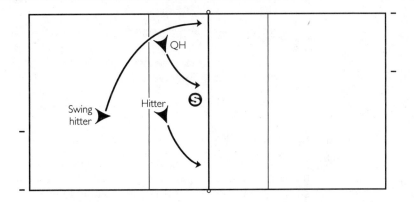

5–1 swing offense:
Multiple options

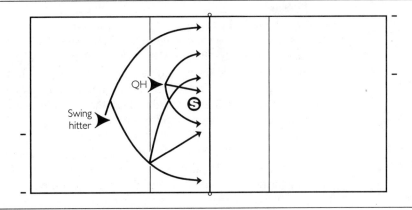

The *swing offense* is a recent innovation in offensive volleyball. It was developed by Doug Beal, the men's gold-medal winning coach for the 1984 Olympics. In the traditional style of attack, the players move perpendicular to the net when attacking. In the swing offense, the players move laterally, then attack either on the perpendicular or at a diagonal angle. This style of offense makes it very difficult for the blockers to detect who will be attacking and which area will be attacked. Because of this, their movements are delayed and they are less effective.

The swing attacker may hide behind the quick hitter and then flare to either side of the court and receive the set. In this offense, the hitters usually call out their attack patterns.

Checklist for Offensive Systems

1. The 6–6 is a system in which every player sets and hits, depending on their positions on the court.
2. The 4–2 is a two-hitter attack. There must be four good hitters and two good setters. The set will nearly always come from the setter in the front line.
3. The 6–2 is a three-hitter attack. There will always be three people who can hit in the front line and one setter who comes up from the back line. All six players must be good hitters and two must be good setters.
4. The 5–1 is a combination of the previous two systems. There must be one great setter and five good hitters.

Calling Plays

At the beginner level, no play may be called. If one is called, it may be nothing more than telling the player who will attack that the ball is coming that way, such as "Here, Joe" or "Marilyn, it's coming to you."

At the intermediate level, the setter will call the zone of the set from which the ball will be attacked. For example, if the set will be to the left front (zone 4), the call would be "Four."

At the advanced levels, there are many possible elements to a call, such as the area of the net, the height of the set, the path of the attacker, the bunching or spreading of the offense, and the coordination of the front- and back-row attacks.

Calling the plays can be done with hand signals or by verbal signals (audibilizing). The play that is called will tell the area of the net to which the set will travel and the relative height of the set above the net. This is done with numbers.

The standard front-row attack areas for volleyball in the United States call for nine areas along the net. Each area is approximately one meter long. The area farthest left is designated as "1," the next area is "2," and so forth up to area "9." This area is always the first element signaled in a play call.

The second element is the relative height of the set. The second number tells number of feet above the net that the set should reach. So a call of "31" would indicate a set into area 3 that would be one foot above the net. A "95" call would be a set five feet above the top of the net into area 9 (the far-right end of the net.)

The back-row attack areas are measured along the three-meter line. The line is divided into four equal corridors designated as (from left to right) A, B, C, and D. For a back-row attack, all that is necessary to know is the area of the attack, so only the letter is called—no number. The setter and hitter will know the necessary height of the set.

Strategies for Coed Volleyball

Because of the rules differences for coed volleyball, some differences in strategy may also exist. Since a woman player can attack the net or block even if playing a back-court position, a woman who is tall or has great jumping ability can be called into the attack more often.

Coed formation

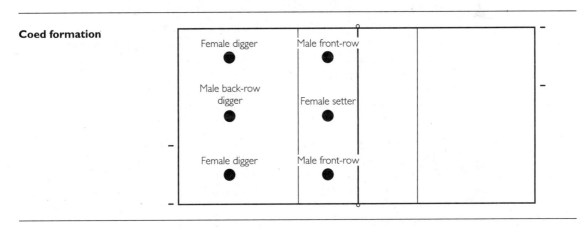

Coed defensive variations

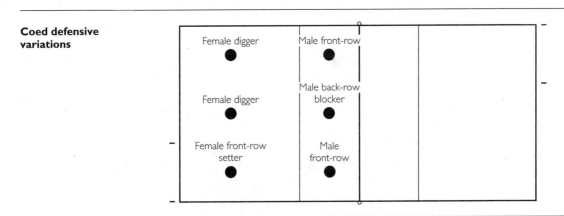

Generally, a man is the best hitter-blocker, so when a man is in the front row he should be switched into the left forecourt as often as possible so that he can be the on-hand hitter.

Just as in any advanced play the setter, who is usually a female, should play the right-back position as often as possible because there is easier access to the net from that point.

Because of the rule that requires that a woman play the ball at least once if it is contacted two or more times, the women players should be positioned as passers or setters. If a man is the designated setter, the women must be passers because a male is nearly always the best attacker.

Drills

1. *The rhythm side out.* This is a continuous service-receive drill in which one team continues to serve and the other continues to receive. The team will rotate on every serve.

2. *Continuous hitter coverage.* This is a drill using a blocking device that will rebound every attacked ball. The attacking team will pass, set, and attack, then play the rebounded ball and repeat the sequence.

3. *Side out with criteria.* (Criteria are standards of success such as five total successful plays prior to rotating, or five successful plays in a row.) The teacher or coach should choose a high level of criteria that is obtainable for the level of players. After meeting a criterion, the team will rotate. The serving team will continue to serve until the teacher or coach calls for a change.

4. *Wash drill.* This is a two-way drill (offense and defense) with each team having an opportunity to score. Team A serves and plays the ball until the rally is over. Team B then serves a ball and plays until the rally is over. If one team wins both rallies, that team earns a point. If each team wins one rally, it is a tie (a "wash"). The teacher can determine the number of points necessary to rotate or to win this drill.

Summary

1. There are several basic offensive systems. They are designated by the number of attackers and the number of setters in the scheme.

2. A 6–6 system is the most common for beginners. In this system each player is a setter or an attacker, depending on their positions on the court during the serve.

3. Intermediate teams may use a 4–2 (four hitters and two setters) system.

4. Advanced teams will use a 6–2 (six attackers, two designated setters) system, or a 5–1 (five attackers, one setter) system.

5. Teams must have formations for serve-receiving and hitter coverage.

11 *Team Defense*

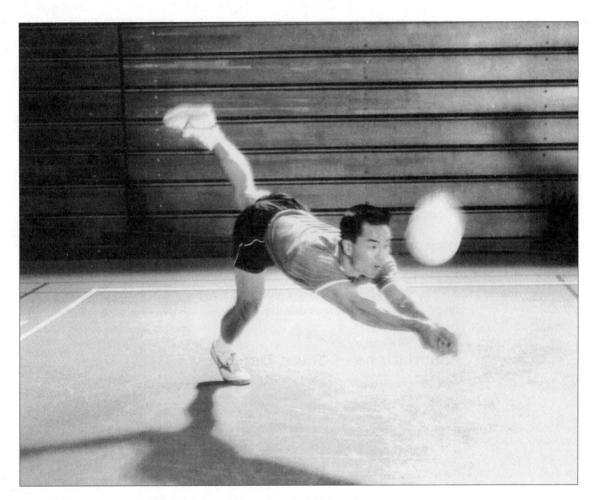

Outline

The major job of the defensive team is to score points. All systems and tactics should be based on this premise. Scoring is accomplished by the blockers (the front-line defense), who terminate attacked balls by penetrating the net and blocking the attack to the floor.

As mentioned in Chapter 8, many teachers and coaches underestimate the importance of training players to technically and tactically block well as individuals, or, more importantly, to block well as a team. Continually terminating attacked balls by knocking them to the floor is very intimidating to the unsuccessful attackers and to the unsuccessful attacking team as a whole. Terminating attacked balls or digging and successfully counterattacking the attack team's balls can often change the rhythm of a game or match.

The second line of defense is comprised of the team members who are not involved in the block. This second line includes the front-row player not participating in the block, who is called the "off blocker."

All defenses should be based on what moves the offense is capable of making and what the defenders are capable of executing. A defensive team should not attempt to do tactically what it cannot do technically. Defenses should, as a rule, coordinate the front-row blockers with the second-line players (those teammates not involved in the block). It is the job of the teacher or coach to determine which defensive systems and tactics are appropriate for the team's personnel to employ in general and against specific opponents.

It is common for young volleyball players to be out of balance in their skill development. Usually the elements of offense (the pass, the set, and the attack) are emphasized more than the elements of defensive play. But teachers and coaches should be aware that volleyball is no different from most other sports—teams with the best defense usually are the most successful teams.

Foundations of Team Defense

Following are some of the foundations of team defense.

Theory:

- Coordinate the second line of defense with the first line.
- Formulate alignments that solidify tip coverage.

Play:

- Players should watch events in this order: the opponent's pass, the setter, the set to its apex, *their own block*, and finally the attacker.
- Dig the ball to the desired target area—preferably to the three-meter line.

Mind set for winning:

- Playing successful team defense (digging, pursuing balls to keep them off the floor, counterattacking) is tough, and success is contagious.

Eye contact sequence for blocking:
1. Passed ball;
2. Setter; 3. Ball set;
4. Attacker

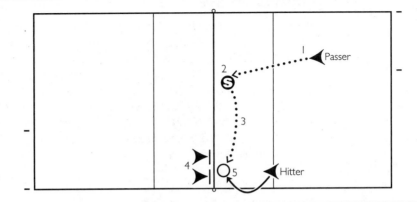

- Teams that are successful should celebrate, or at least acknowledge, in good sportsmanship style, their victories.

The *theory and standards of performance* should be developed in the following areas:

Theory:

- Changing the defensive scheme while thinking aggressively makes the offense respond to and worry about your systems, tactics, and personnel.
- Successful counterattacking is essential at the elite levels of volleyball. (The USA men's teams in the 1984 and 1988 Olympics won the gold medals primarily because they were significantly better than the competition in counterattacking.)

Technique:

- The ball should be played with both feet planted, and with two arms on the ball as often as possible.

Mind set for winning:

- High-level teams must develop an aggressive team approach to the work ethic on defense.
- A team must adopt an enthusiasm for pursuing all balls that are spiked, deflected, or tipped.
- Communication with teammates must be maintained during play situations such as the standard dig-set-hit sequence and other spontaneous situations.
- "Swinging to score" while counterattacking makes the defensive team more aggressive.
- Adopt the motto: "If we have the ball, the opponent pays."

Defensive Systems

The major job of the defense is to offset or neutralize the spiking attack of the offensive team. This can be done from any of several alignments. While beginners need to concentrate on playing only one defense, intermediate and advanced players need more options to stop the more varied attacks at the higher levels of play.

The defensive theory begins with the number of people involved in attempting to block the ball. If the attacking team does not have a chance to spike, no blockers are required. Some situations require only one blocker, some two, and some three blockers.

Progression of Defenses

The *"W" defense with no blocker* is a defense for beginners who do not know how to spike.

W defense

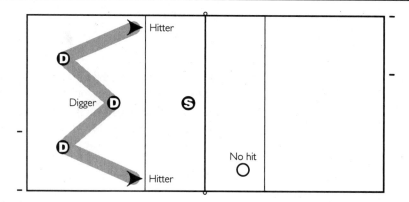

One-blocker defense

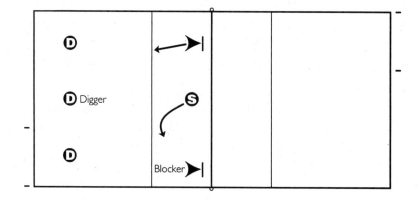

The *"W" defense with one blocker* at the net is a scheme for beginners whose attackers may have the ability to drive the ball down into the defender's court. One blocker is designated to be at the point of attack and prepared to block the ball if necessary.

The *up defense* brings a player up from the back row to cover behind the block for any tipped, offspeed, or deflected balls. It is common practice to bring up the center back-row player (zone 6) or the setter, but any back-row player can be the designated "up" player. Some teachers or coaches have their weakest defensive player up because they feel it gets that person out of the way.

Up defense:
Middle digger up

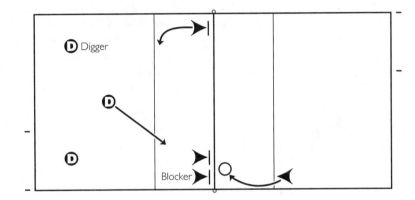

The "up" player gets behind the block and straddles the three-meter line. It is obvious from the diagrams that the defensive player in the "up" position does not have to move much and that both the tip and the perimeter are covered. A team can use a digger or setter as the up player.

Most beginning and intermediate teams use an up defense, as do most advanced teams.

Setter-up defense

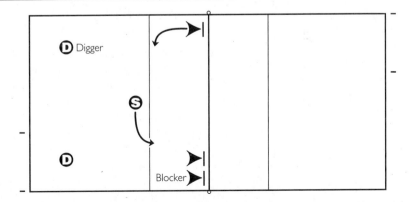

Back defense:
Right side set

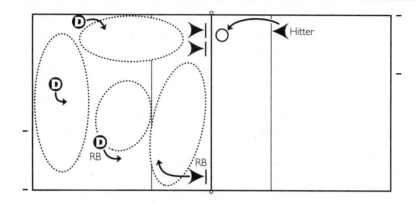

Quick hitter defense

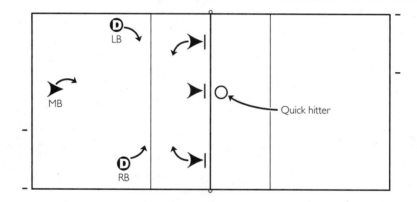

The *back* or *perimeter defense* is a defense used primarily against good hitting teams. The weaknesses of this defense are that the middle of the court is vulnerable (in theory, no ball should be hit into this area) and the fact that the line digger on the side of the attacker and the off blocker (the blocker on the opposite side) have dual responsibility for the driven ball and the tipped ball. This dual responsibility often finds these two players moving or charging in as the ball is attacked.

The center back in this defense should not necessarily stay in the exact center back part of the court on every play. Instead, the position of the center back should be based on the abilities of the blockers and the tactics and tendencies of the various attackers.

The off blocker's responsibility is the sharp angled spike or the tip inside the block. The back-row angle digger is usually positioned to see the ball and the attacker. This player should not be behind the blockers unless it is by design. Often this player is sent to the corner to retrieve deep-corner attacks.

This defense can be used at any level, but requires considerable practice time or experience to cover the offspeed situations that may arise.

The *rotate defense* is a simple but solid defense. The line digger on the side of the court where the attack originates moves up and is responsible for the tip. The center back rotates to the corner vacated by the line digger. The other back-row player moves to the opposite corner. The key player in this defense is the off blocker, who must react to the set, then quickly get to the primary digging position before the attacker contacts the ball.

The two back-row players have flexibility to adjust the court balance for attackers with strong tendencies. Some teams rotate for attacks to one side but not to the other side.

Rotate left side set

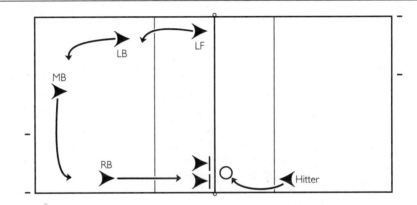

Rotate to right side set

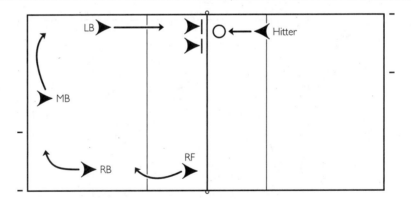

The *slide defense* has the off blocker sliding over behind the block to cover the tip, the offspeed hit, and the deflected ball. The strong point of this defense is that the back-court players have only one responsibility—to play the driven balls. The off blocker (in theory) has all tips.

Some teachers, coaches, and players see this defense as hindering a strong counterattacking transition. If the slide blocker happens to be the strongest

Slide defense

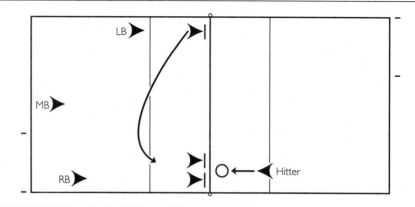

front-row attacker, that person may not be in position to counterattack. (The argument to counter this criticism is that the game should be played one play at a time, so counterattacking does not receive a higher priority for the first play than court coverage.)

The *switch defense* is used by some high-level teams as their high set defense. For example, in the case of a high set to the offensive left-front attacker, the left-back defensive player moves over and up to take the tip responsibility. This play can be automatic or audibilized by experienced players. This defense enables the off blocker to be in good position for counterattacking.

Switching to defensive positions from serve

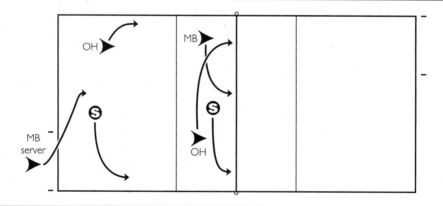

The *free ball defense* is used when the ball is not spiked and a block is therefore not needed. When defending a free ball, the setter moves to the center-front position while the other players resume the W service reception formation. The blockers back up, the middle back moves back slightly, and the diggers move farther into the court.

Free ball

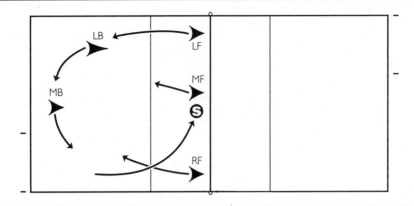

Drills

1. *Positioning.* The teacher stands on a box or table and hits balls to the areas of defensive responsibilities. Players play out the ball. This can be used with any defense.
2. *Situation defense.* The defensive team has to react to a traditional attack, a free ball, or a down-the-line shot. The coach or teacher can do this by tossing the ball to an offensive player and commanding that player to perform the maneuver that was called, such as a bump or spike.
3. *The 8 vs. 4.* The teacher or coach continually tosses the ball over the net to the offensive team so that they can run their offensive combinations. The offense needs eight kills to rotate, and the defensive team needs four points to rotate. The scoring can be adjusted to keep this drill in competitive balance. This is an excellent drill because it gives the defense numerous opportunities to respond in game-related situations.
4. *Offense vs. defense wash.* See offensive drills in Chapter 10.

 Checklist for Team Defense

1. The front-row players nearest the attack form the block. (For an attack from the right side of the defense, it would be the right-front and center-front players.)
2. Defensive players should watch, in order: the pass, the setter, the set, their own block, and finally the attacker.
3. All defensive schemes should include responsibility for tip coverage.

Summary

1. The defense must attempt to score.
2. Beginners usually play only one defensive alignment, but more advanced teams need several types of alignments to be able to stop the various attacks and strengths of their opponents.
3. The common defenses are the W with no blocker, the W with one blocker, the up, the back, the rotate, the slide, the switch, and the free ball.

12   *Team Transitions*

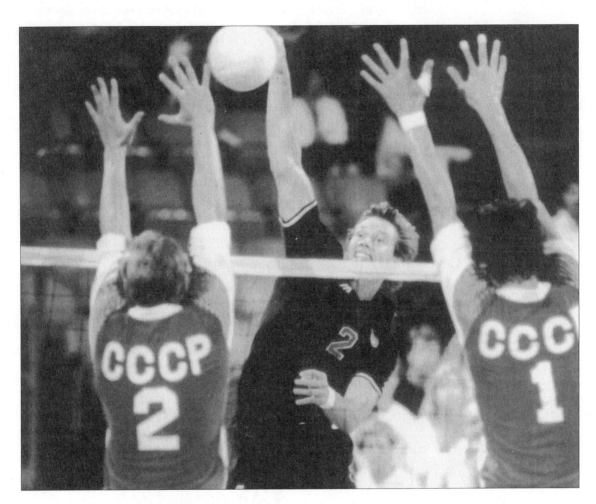

Outline

Transitions from service receiving to hitter coverage, from offense to defense, and from defense to offense must be done quickly and correctly in order to maximize the success of the team. Teams that have exceptional talent but that don't make effective transitions look disjointed and will not play up to their capabilities, whereas teams with average talent that make good transitions can look like well-oiled machines.

A team should be in either a scoring mode (if it has the serve) or in a side-out mode (if it is trying to regain the serve). The difference is that in a scoring mode the team should be more aggressive in order to gain the point, and in a side-out mode the play is more conservative so that the team does not give up a point.

Service Receiving to Attack and Hitter Coverage

When the ball is passed after the serve, the players move forward. As the ball is set, all players "read" the set and immediately react to the set ball. During the set, the non-attacking players move to their positions in the inner cup or the outer cup of the hitter coverage. (See Chapter 10 for a further discussion of offensive moves.)

Offense to Defense

All players immediately react to the attacked ball. The front-row players move immediately to their blocking or spike protection responsibilities. The back-row players move immediately to their defensive responsibilities. They must get back quickly so that their teammates will be in front of them. If they accomplish this, the play will probably be made in front of them. Wherever a player is positioned on the court, it is essential that he or she be stationary, not moving, at the moment that the ball is being hit.

Volleyball is a "forward" game—movements should be made forward. The only reason to move backward is to be in a position to be able to move forward

Transition from offense to defense

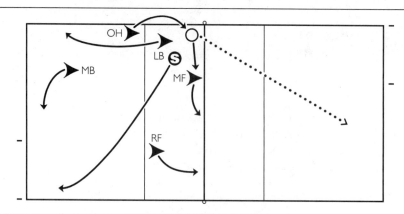

when the moment comes to play the ball. Note, however, that the setter moves back to the designed defensive position or a blocking position. Many setters stay close to the net and watch the game, failing to switch to defense.

Defense to Offense

All players watch the path of the ball and react accordingly. The transition of the blockers is very important. First they move quickly to the three-meter line. Once the ball is passed, the back-row players cover the hitter by moving into their defensive positions. This is the key—the ball and their teammates must be in front of them. The setter and non-attacking front-row players move into their positions immediately after the set.

Transition from defense to offense

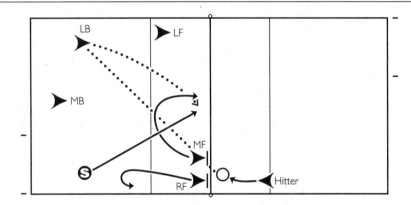

There are three types of transition opportunities when changing from defense to offense: the standard defensive counterattack, the free ball, and the down ball.

The *standard defensive counterattack* is executed when the defense plays an attacked ball effectively, resulting in an opportunity to spike. The setter release occurs immediately when the ball is not attacked to the setter's defensive area. In this case, the setter moves to the designated offensive area. If the ball is played to the setter's area, he or she must play it.

Free ball coverage is used when the opponents are not able to attack with a spike. This is generally an advantage for the team taking the offense. The W formation, used in serve reception, is an effective free ball alignment. The major difference is that the setter is allowed to play in the preferred setting position and does not have to take a back-court responsibility, as might be required in defending a serve.

The setter release occurs when it is certain that the ball will not be attacked. The setter must then move to the designated offensive position. The other defensive players must balance the court when the setter releases.

The *down ball* occurs when the blockers have prepared to block, then decide that it is not necessary to block because the opponents cannot drive the ball down into their court. This can occur when the attacker slips or mistimes the set. The blockers at the point of attack stay adjacent to the net, the off blocker moves to the defensive assignment, and the back-row players move one meter into the court.

The setter release is similar to the standard defense—the setter cannot release until it is certain that the ball will be played by a teammate. The eye contact sequence of the defenders is to watch the setter, the set, their team's blockers, and then the hitter. It is not necessary to hear the blockers say "down" (meaning that they will stay down on the ground and not attempt to block the ball).

Giving direction in all transition situations is the responsibility of the setter. If the ball is played in a manner in which the setter cannot set the ball, the setter must identify the individual who is to set the ball and the best location in which to make the set. The experienced setter can also give direction to the attackers prior to and during the transition.

The passers are the primary ball-control players. They should play as many of the transition balls as possible.

Switching in transition should be done only when there is time to accomplish it. For example, a left-front attacker who has swung to the right to hit may have to remain in that spot for a portion of the rally until there is time to switch back to the left front.

Common errors in making transitions include:

- Not having a mind set focused on scoring
- Stagnant counterattacks
- Failure to use the entire net and all attack options
- Poor communication on the court

 Checklist for the Individual in Transition

1. Know whether you are in a scoring (aggressive) mode or a side-out (conservative) mode in your transitions.
2. Watch the ball.
3. React immediately to the position of the ball and to the attack.
4. Be stationary, not moving, when the ball is attacked.
5. Volleyball is a "forward" game—you move back only to be ready to move forward to play the ball.

Drills

1. Service receiving to hitter coverage. This is a continuous hitter coverage drill. See Chapter 10 for a full explanation.

2. Offense to defense. Starting with an offensive combination (pass, set, hit), a dug ball is played out. If the spike is killed, the teacher immediately throws a ball to the defensive team or the offensive team.

3. Defense to offense. Start in a defensive alignment with one, two, or three blockers and the remaining players in their correct defensive positions. The teacher or coach gives the offensive team a free ball, tosses a ball to the attacker for a down ball situation (the ball cannot be driven down into the opponent's court), or tosses a ball for a traditional attack.

4. Repetitive transition. Both the front rows are at the net and the teacher or coach tosses a ball to either side. That side then makes the transition from defense to offense.

Summary

1. Making the transition quickly from offense to defense or defense to offense is essential to a team's achieving its maximum efficiency.

2. When switching from defense to offense, the blockers must quickly retreat to the three-meter line and be ready to set, if necessary, in order to counterattack.

3. When switching from offense to defense, the blockers must be alert to the ball and be ready to move toward the opponent's attacker as the set is made.

4. The major transition situations in volleyball are from serve receiving to hitter coverage, from offense to defense, and from defense to offense.

5. The transition from defense to offense must take into account whether the team will play a standard defense, a free ball defense, or a down ball defense.

13　*Outdoor Volleyball*

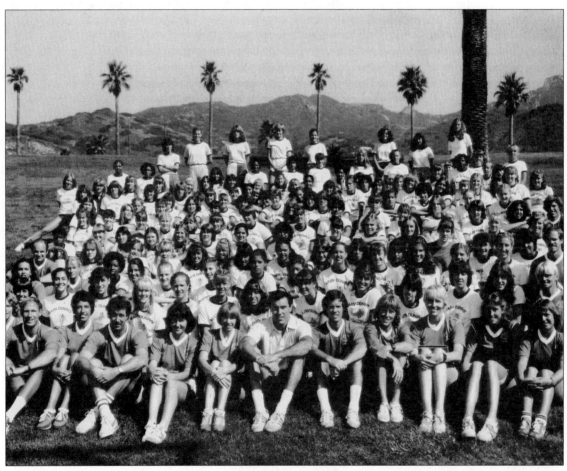

Coach Dunphy with participants in volleyball camp at Pepperdine University

Outline

The United States Volleyball Association sanctions many levels of volleyball in the United States—from the Olympic team to junior-level play and from high school and YMCA to the professional ranks. Other associations sanction other levels of the game.

While different levels of play may have different rules (such as international, women's college, or high school federations), they are all sanctioned by the umbrella organization of the United States Volleyball Association.

Professional play is rapidly growing in both the two-player beach game (either men or women) and the six-player indoor games (both men and women). Sports television has increased interest for the fans and the prizes for the players.

Youth and junior play is the fastest-growing and largest area of volleyball today. There are divisions for players aged up to 13, for those 14 and 15, and for those 16 and 17.

The *YMCA* has been involved in volleyball since its inception, because the game was invented at a YMCA. Nearly every YMCA and YWCA has a volleyball program. They also hold their own national championships.

Corporate leagues are an expanding area of volleyball interest. Some companies have their own courts, while others rent or schedule courts at schools or public parks.

City leagues exist in most cities. The local recreation department will generally be able to inform you as to when and where the leagues will play. Check on specific requirements such as liability or health insurance, a physical exam, and entry fees.

Types of Outdoor Volleyball

Outdoor volleyball is a common recreational game. Whether it is played at the company picnic or in a professional beach tournament, it is enjoyable and exciting.

Beach volleyball has been played since at least the 1940s. It is played with two people on each team: two men, two women, or mixed. Because it is played on the sand, the players can dive without fear of being hurt, and because they play the same 30 by 60 foot court dimensions as indoor players, they must be in good physical condition.

The Professional Beach Volleyball Tour, with its newspaper and television coverage, has created both nationwide and worldwide attention. The international professional beach tour has been a great success with fans both at the beach and on TV. The recent addition of sand doubles volleyball as an Olympic sport has greatly increased its visibility and the interest of the beach-going public. We now see sand volleyball courts everywhere from the beaches at Venice, California, to the valleys of Norway.

Playing beach volleyball is not limited to courts along the oceans and lakes of the country. For example, tournaments such as those in Denver, Vail, or Aspen, Colorado have used sand courts for more than 30 years. Many colleges have also built sand courts. The beach has come to the midlands! The sport was just too exciting to be limited to the beaches of Southern California.

Rule Differences for Outdoor Volleyball

There are some differences between indoor and outdoor volleyball. For example, the outdoor ball is inflated with less air pressure so the wind does not have as much effect on it is it would on the indoor ball.

Some of the *rules differences* for outdoor volleyball are major; they include:

- Two people per team with no substitutes allowed.
- A match is a single game of 15 points. (This can be changed by a tournament director. Eleven-point games may be played.)
- Players will switch sides every five points (for example, at a three to two or four to one score) in a 15-point game and every four points in an 11-point game.
- The ball may be served from anywhere behind the end line and between the sidelines extended.
- Outdoor players are allowed to stay in contact with a set longer than indoor players without being called for a "lift." But outdoor officiating does not allow for a set ball to spin; if it does, it is called a "double hit."
- The ball may be contacted with any part of the body.
- Either a blocked ball or a hard-driven ball can be contacted multiple times in succession during one attempt to play the ball.
- A player may move under the net as long as an opponent is not impeded.
- A player can block any ball crossing over the net, including a serve.
- When a player intentionally hits a two-hand overhead pass into the opponent's court, that player's shoulders should be squared up to the ball's line of flight.

Some minor differences include:

- The net height is 7 feet 11 5/8 inches for men and 7 feet 4 1/8 inches for women.
- A coin toss determines which team will choose side or serve.
- The serve must pass over the net between the poles.
- The teammate of the server must be within the court and motionless during the serve.
- The server's partner must grant the opposition a clear view of the ball during the serve and, if asked to move, to open a visual path, must comply.
- Each player will serve continuously until there is a side out. On the next service opportunity the partner will serve.
- If a player serves out of order, he or she is allowed to continue serving for the duration of that service. There is no penalty for serving out of order; however, the partner will serve the next series after the side out.

Grass volleyball uses the same rules for doubles as beach volleyball. When a team has six players, indoor rules are used. The next section deals specifically with the rules of contact in outdoor volleyball.

Rules of Contact for Outdoor Volleyball

The following are rules of contact in outdoor volleyball:

- A player may touch the ball with any part of the body.
- A player may have successive contacts with the ball during a single attempt to make the team's first contact with the ball, provided that the fingers are not used to direct the ball.
- The ball must be contacted cleanly and not held; this means that a player may not lift, push, catch, carry, or throw the ball.
- An exception to the preceding rule is allowed in two- and three-person games during the defensive play of a hard-driven ball, which is an attack-hit or blocked ball traveling at the high rate of speed (as judged by the referee). In that case, the ball may be momentarily lifted or pushed, providing that the attempt is one continuous motion and the player does not change the direction of his or her motion while contacting the ball.
- Contact of the ball with two hands, using the fingers to direct the ball, is a set. A player may set the ball in any direction toward his or her team's court, provided that the ball is contacted simultaneously by both the player's hands and does not visibly come to rest.
- Rotation of the ball after the set may indicate a held ball or multiple contacts during the set, but in itself is not a fault.
- A legal set directed toward a teammate that unintentionally crosses the net is not a fault, regardless of the player's body position. Intent is judged by the referee.
- In a two- or three-person game, if the ball is intentionally set into the opponent's court, the player must contact the ball above his or her shoulders and must direct the ball perpendicular to the direction his or her shoulders are facing.
- In two-, three-, or four-person games, when a player contacts the ball with one hand, it must be cleanly hit with the heel or palm of the hand (a roll shot); with straight, locked fingertips (a cobra); with knurled fingers (a camel toe); or with the back of the hand from the wrist to the knuckles. One-handed placement or redirection of the ball with the fingers (a dink or one-hand tip) is a fault.

Considerations for Outdoor Volleyball

In *doubles*, hand signals are used to designate the area of the court the block is expected to take. If playing in the sand, the sand reduces the height to which a spiker can jump, so the set must be closer to the net. (This makes it easier to block.) The blocker's partner must know where the spiker is likely to hit the ball, then cover that area.

In the *three-player* game, anyone can spike or block. One player usually blocks while the other two are diggers.

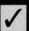 *Checklist for Doubles Rules Differences*

1. Players switch sides every five points in a 15-point game.
2. No open-handed tips are allowed.
3. If passing the ball over the net, the player must face the direction of the hit.
4. A player may pass under the net as long as there is no interference with the opponents.
5. The serve can be from anywhere behind the end line.
6. The ball can be played with any part of the body.

With *four players*, the server is a back-row player and is not allowed to spike or block. Usually only one player is designated as the primary setter.

With *five players*, three are usually designated as front-court players and two as back-court players.

A team with *six players* uses regular international rules, but the digging rules are often relaxed a bit and the ball is allowed to stay in contact an instant longer than would be permissible in the indoor game.

The Effects of Nature on Outdoor Play

The *sun* becomes a major factor when playing defense or receiving the serve. The high serve (sky ball) or high attacking shot, which forces the opponents to look into the sun to play the ball, can be very effective.

The *wind* is such an important factor that a team may choose "side" rather than "serve" in order to obtain the side of the court that faces the incoming wind. The wind blowing into the server helps to force the served ball down and keep it in the court. This is particularly true in a top-spin serve, which is forced rapidly downward by the wind. The floater serve into a moderate wind will also be more likely to hold the ball up, then let it drop nearly straight down.

The wind can be a disadvantage to the team hitting with the wind. A floater serve is often carried outside the court. In fact, any deep shot may well be carried out of bounds.

A cross-wind can aid a spin serve if the player can spin the ball into the wind. For example, a right-handed server with a counterclockwise rotation (server follows through to the right of the ball) will curve the ball left. A wind blowing to the left will accentuate the spin and may give it a curved trajectory two or three times greater than the spin would have imparted on a calm day. Similarly, a right-hander following through to the left of the ball, giving the ball a clockwise movement, will gain additional curvature if the wind is blowing from left to right.

Any wind also has a profound effect on every pass and set. For this reason, the ball should be played lower to reduce this variable.

Hit and block at the beach

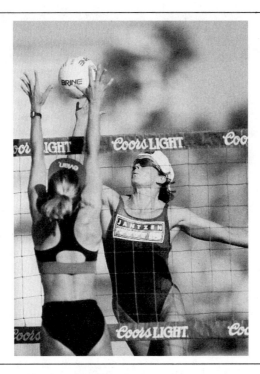

Beach or Doubles Volleyball Play

If you think indoor six-person volleyball is a great sport, try it in the sand with just you and a partner. On a top-level indoors team, you need one or two major skills—setting, hitting, passing, or blocking, along with serving. But on the beach you must be a master of every skill. It's just you and your partner. Not only are more and better skills needed, but doubles requires much better conditioning—and if you are playing in the sand, those legs better be in shape.

If you are a weak passer or hitter, you can expect the serve to come to you every time. If you can't set well, you can bet that your opponents will make certain that you do most of the setting.

Serving

Your serving technique will be pretty much the same on the beach as it is on an indoor hardcourt. However, the softer ball (with its lower inflation) and the wind force you to hit a bit harder on some serves. The wind may also affect your toss, especially if you use a jump serve. Your toss may need to be lower to reduce the wind's effect.

On the beach, your serving tactics will need the most adapting from your indoor style. The heavier ball, the wind, the sun, and the strengths or weak-

Jump serve

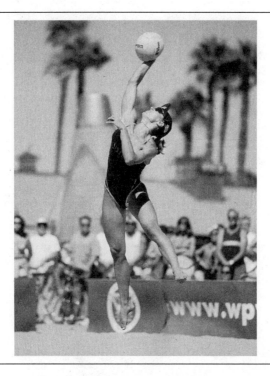

nesses of your opponents will greatly increase your options. For example, if the sun is nearly overhead or high and slightly behind you, a skyball may be a good serve. The sun will obscure the ball from your opponents while the wind will probably do tricks with the ball. The skyball is generally served underhand—preferably with no spin.

It is essential to make your opponents move. You don't want to give them an easy pass. Serve to the person you want to hit—or the weakest passer. What are your opponents' weaknesses? Are they indecisive about who takes serves down the middle? Does one of them have problems with high or low serves? Is one of your opponents out of shape? If so, make him or her work—pass, jump, and hit.

If you get your choice of side for beginning the match, take the wind in your face. You will have a better chance of getting your strong serves in and your hits will have the benefit of the wind pushing them down.

Passing

Let's start with passing. If you're playing outside, especially at the beach, you can expect some wind—sometimes *lots* of wind; it will make the ball do tricks that even the server can't predict. And that high "rainmaker" serve can confuse the passer as it drifts from one sideline to the other in its descent. Then the hard serve, like a jump serve, forces you to be able to move quickly in any

Checklist for Serving in Beach Volleyball

1. With the sun high consider a skyball.
2. Serve to the weakest passer or to the person you want to hit the attacking hit.
3. Against the wind you can serve harder.
4. With a cross-wind, think of spinning the ball to increase the arc of your serve. Your follow-through will be on the wind side of the ball.
5. Serve closer to the wind side to avoid the possibility of the wind carrying the ball out.

Dig in the sand

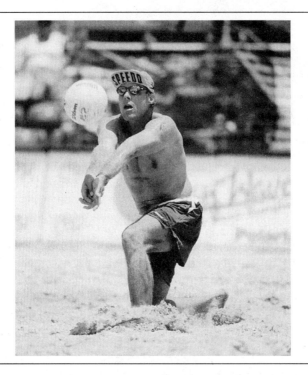

direction. For this reason, your ready position needs to be lower and well balanced.

Try to get both forearms on the ball with every pass. Use a one-handed dig only as a last resort—there is too great a chance that a one-handed pass will be misdirected.

If a spike comes high and hard, you can use an overhand dig. Open your fingers wide and let the ball hit your palms and fingers at the same time. If the ball stays too long on your hand, you will be called for a "throw."

Your target is also different when you play in the sand: you should hit straight in front of you. That way your partner can anticipate where to move. Set the ball back five or six feet from the net so there is no chance to hit the net with your pass and your partner has room to move.

Setting

Try to make your set overhand. Although there are many good setters who bump set, the overhand set gives most players better control. Then set where you know your partner wants it—high, low, middle, wide. You're not going to fool your opponents—they know who is going to hit the ball and they can see where that hit will take place.

If your partner is out of position, having had to go deep or wide, he or she should tell you where to set the ball: "high middle," "high right," or "behind" are examples of calls that might be made. Gauge the wind; if it is blowing at you, set it harder. If it is blowing in the direction of your set, don't aim as far as you would indoors—the breeze will take care of the rest. If the topspin of the ball is spinning away, the ball will go farther, so reduce your thrust.

Hitting

It is much more difficult to jump out of the sand to spike than to jump off a hard surface. Because of this, many teams play both defenders back and hope to be able to cover. As players have become taller and have increased their jumping ability, it has become necessary to send one person up as a blocker. If you're going to spike, you now have to angle around or over the block.

If you are playing against a team that sends a blocker, you need to be able to hit the corners. You don't necessarily have to hit as hard as you do indoors. You just have to "hit it where they ain't." Think placement, not power. Look to the corners. If you pop the ball over the blocker, deep and away from the other player, you have a great chance for a winner—and even if you don't win a point, at least it's a very difficult pass for your opponent. But make sure you keep every hit in bounds; there is no sense in giving away an unearned point.

Keep every approach, jump, and hit position the same on every shot. Only at the time of the hit do you hit with power, cut, dink, or angle your shot. If you disguise your intentions, your opponents can't read your shot and move before you have actually hit the ball.

The *dink* is hit by slowing down your arm motion and your wrist snap at the last instant. If there is no one near the net, you can softly clear the net and have the ball land in front of your opponents. If there is a blocker, aim higher, deeper and away from the other defender.

The *cut* is a difficult shot to master. Aim the ball just over the net and seven to eight feet away so that the blocker doesn't have a chance to touch it. The cut must be hit softly enough to fall in bounds. Hit one to three inches to the side

Big hit

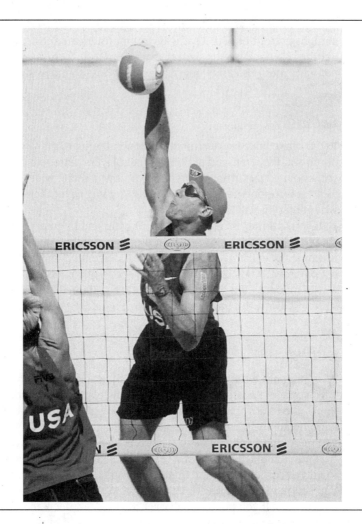

of the ball. Your wrist will go over and around the ball to put spin on it and direct it sideways. You can cut to either side of the blocker.

Deeper shots to either sideline, a deep line or a deep angle, are hit harder but still with control. Hit the middle of the ball as with any spike. Depending on how accurate you are, you can aim three to eight feet in on the imaginary diagonal running from either back corner. If you are hitting from the front corner of your court, you have 30 feet down the line and 42.4 feet to the other corner. The odds favor the deeper hit if it is there.

Better players are able to take a quick look as they make their approach to hit—but their expert partners will probably set the ball just about where expected. The lower the level of play, the more variables, so keep consistent. Try to avoid errors rather than playing "hit and hope."

Hit and block

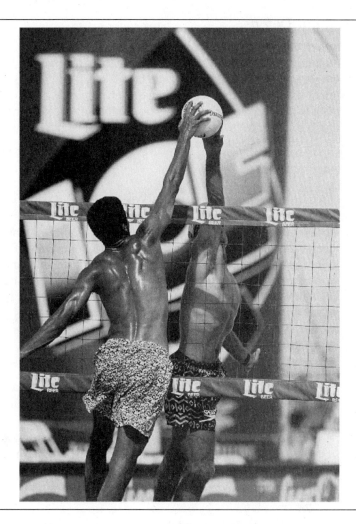

Blocking

Blockers can go over the net, just as in the indoor game. Stay in front of the hitter, then move to the angle you have told your partner you will defend—left, straight ahead, or right. (Your partner will defend the remaining area.) Take your ready position a foot to a foot and a half off the net. You don't want to get so close that you will "net," nor so far away that you can't reach over. While a few pros signal after the pass is made, most people are more secure making their signals before the serve. It is much clearer, and you have time to register what you are going to do.

Team Defense

When you are serving, you can often set up a tactical approach to playing the first defensive opportunity. The server can tell the partner where the serve will go and where to block, or fake a block. Moves that change the defensive alignment with a fake block on the angle, then an actual block of the down-the-line shot with the digger faking covering the line, then defending the angle—this kind of sequence gives servers a chance to make the offensive team uneasy and perhaps less effective.

Team Offense

You and your partner will generally divide the court in half. However, you may both move a foot or two in any direction, depending on where the serves have been successful. Move back if deep serves are effective, up if the ball is diving, right if the server is consistent hitting your right sideline, and so on.

You also need to talk. The setter should be able to see the blocker and the digger immediately after the set. He can then tell the hitter to "hit" if there is no blocker, "cut" if the digger is deep, and so on.

Summary

1. Volleyball is becoming increasingly popular. The media is increasing its coverage of the game, and players find the game exciting.
2. Beach or sand volleyball is played with two players per side. The rules are somewhat different than the international rules for indoor volleyball.
3. Variations of the game include two-, three-, four-, and six-person teams.
4. Outdoor volleyball strategy must consider the effects of the sun and wind on the way the ball will respond, and how these forces of nature will affect the opponents.
5. You can use the sun and the wind to put your opponents at a disadvantage, increasing the effectiveness of your serves.
6. Strategy becomes a more intimate part of the game because there are only two players involved on each side.

14 *Common Injuries In Volleyball*

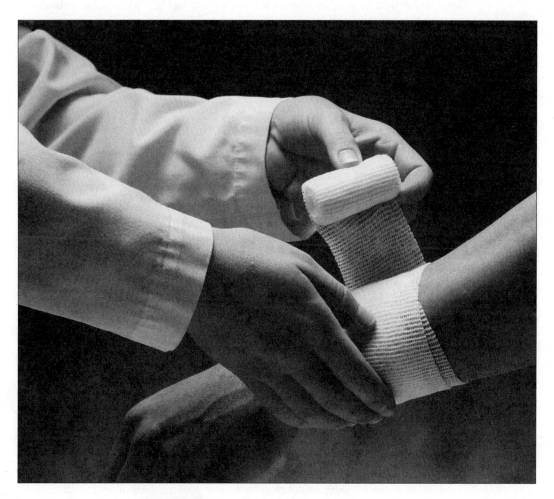

Outline

every sport has injury problems: some of them are "overuse" types of injuries such as those seen in joggers' ankles, lower legs, and knees, while others are acute injuries such as when a basketball player sprains an ankle. In volleyball, finger injuries have gone down over the years due to more passing with the forearms, but ankle sprains have increased because people are jumping higher and more often in spiking and blocking. And allowing the jumpers to land on or over the center line has increased these injuries even more.

Passing, digging, and setting are quite safe, but blocking and spiking increase the risk of hand, shoulder, knee, and ankle problems. Over 60 percent of all injuries are due to jumping or landing. As you would expect, playing on a soft surface such as sand greatly reduces the number of injuries. In fact, there are 80 percent fewer injuries on sand than on a hard court.

When Injuries Occur

Scientific studies of injuries do not report a consistent incidence of problems because some studies are done with elite players in tournaments, while others are done in physical education classes. But we can surmise from the studies that there are more injuries at the beginning of a season than later—due to poor conditioning and poor skills; and that there are more injuries as the intensity of the game increases, such as in tournaments. There is a higher rate of injuries during games than during practice time. Generally speaking, volleyball is a very safe game, but as spiking, blocking, and diving for digs have become more commonplace, injury rates have risen over the years due to this more aggressive play.

Types of Volleyball Injuries

With advanced and elite volleyball players, we are finding more *overuse* injuries. The continual jumping and landing of hitters and blockers can result in "jumper's knee" (an inflammation of the tendon that holds the kneecap), as well as cruciate ligament tears inside the knee and inflamed tendons where the muscles used in jumping are attached to the thigh and leg bones. About 40 percent of elite players have complained of knee injuries from overuse.

Hitters are more likely to develop shoulder problems both from the stretching of muscles in the upper back (the infraspinatus muscle) and from the force developed in the rotator cuff muscles in the spike and the serve.

For most players, *acute* injuries are more common. The most common types of acute injuries are sprained ankles or wrists, jammed fingers, or twisted knees. Hand injuries account for about half of the reported injuries in school classes. Sprained ankles are second, with an incidence of about 20 percent. At the higher levels of play, injuries to the ankles and knees are more likely, with half of all injuries being to the lower extremities. Some studies show that the

Severe ligament sprain

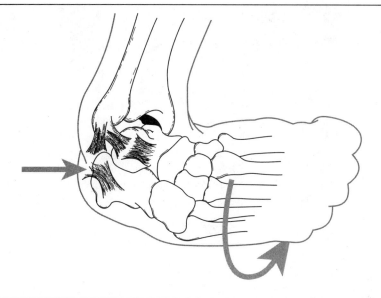

ankles are more often injured, while others show that knees are more often the problem.

Head and upper-body problems are not a major type of volleyball injury. However, a broken nose or extreme twists of the neck (cervical vertebrae) or lower back (lumbar vertebrae) do occur. Less than 10 percent of all volleyball injuries are to the trunk and head.

Arm, shoulder, and hand injuries make up about 30 percent of volleyball injuries. As mentioned, the overhand actions of serving and hitting can cause some problems to the tendons and muscles of the shoulder joint. Elbows don't seem to be a problem, but a few cases of forearm problems have been reported. The wrist and hand are often problems, however. There are eight bones in the wrist with five hand bones attaching to them, as well as two thumb bones and three in each finger, giving a large number of places where a fracture or a sprain (overstretching/rupturing of the ligaments that hold one bone to another) can occur. About 22 percent of injuries are to the fingers, with another 22 percent to the thumbs. Blocking is the major cause of finger and thumb injuries.

Research in Italy at all levels of play has indicated that the floater serve and spike both stretch nerves that may eventually become painful. A major problem in both techniques is a weakness in the muscles that rotate the upper arm in the shoulder[1]. These muscles can be strengthened by doing the rotator cuff exercises provided in Chapter 16.

---

[1]A. DeCarli, "Suprascapular nerve injury in volleyball: The mechanics of the floater serve," presentation at the World Congress of Sports Medicine, May 31, 1998.

✓   *Checklist for Safety*

1. Wear pads to protect your knees or elbows if they are in danger of injuries from the position you play.
2. Wear ankle braces to prevent ankle sprains.
3. Do rotator cuff exercises to reduce shoulder problems from serving and hitting.
4. Do leg exercises to condition the leg muscles for the maximum efforts they must accomplish during practices and games.
5. Consider the use of orthotics and/or cushioned heel cups if you have foot problems.

Leg, ankle, and foot injuries are common in any sport involving running and jumping. Basketball and volleyball players as well as high and long jumpers are prone to the same types of knee, lower leg, and ankle overuse injuries. However, acute injuries in volleyball can also occur in these areas when the knee is twisted or hit from the side or the ankle is twisted during landing. As you might expect, blocking and spiking are the activities during which most lower-leg acute injuries occur.

Small tears in the tendon that surrounds the kneecap, due to both jumping and landing, create a major overuse problem. Shock-absorbing shoes, foot orthotics, and ankle braces can reduce the incidence of such injuries by 80 percent[2]. Strength exercises for the hips, knees, and ankles are also effective preventers of injuries; see Chapter 16.

Risk of Injury

There are gender differences in the occurrence of injuries. Male players are more likely to acquire "jumper's knee" (an injury to the patellar tendon) and shoulder injuries, while female players are more at risk for fractures and knee ligament injuries.

Even though beach volleyball is generally safer than indoor play, sand players are more susceptible to Achilles tendon problems.

---

[2]A. Gollhofer, "Biomechanics of jumping in volleyball: Minimizing the risk"; and R. Bahr, "Ankle sprains: Injury mechanisms and preventive strategies," presentations at the World Congress of Sports Medicine, May 31, 1998.

Checklist for Reducing Injuries

1. Use ankle stabilizers to reduce ankle sprains.
2. Use knee pads to reduce knee injuries from hitting the floor.
3. Play on dry wooden floors. (High-friction or non-skid surfaces such as concrete increase risk as do low-friction or slippery or wet surfaces.)
4. Strengthen the muscles of the legs and shoulders through the use of resistance exercises.

The risk of injuries in volleyball is increased in the following conditions:

- When players are older; older women have more overuse injuries, while older men have more acute injuries.
- Elite players have twice the injury rate of less accomplished players.
- The highest level of injury risk is for young players during their growth spurt.
- If the player has had injuries earlier from volleyball or another sport, there is a risk of re-injury.
- Poor hitting or jumping and landing technique results in an increased risk of injury.
- Injuries can occur if there is an imbalance of muscle strength; for example, if the muscles in the front of the thigh (quadriceps) are much stronger than those in the back of the thighs (hamstrings).
- If the level of competition is higher, the pressure can result in injuries.
- It is more dangerous to play on concrete than on wood or linoleum floors.
- Playing on different surfaces (such as concrete or wood) increases the injury risk over playing on just one surface regularly.

Summary

1. Most sports have some potential for injury.
2. Injuries can often be prevented by using proper techniques and by effective strengthening of the muscles.
3. Protective pads, orthotics and braces; particularly ankle stabilizers, can greatly reduce the risk of injury.
4. Jumping and overhand hitting (spiking or serving) are among the most common volleyball movements resulting in injuries.

15 Aerobic and Anaerobic Conditioning for Volleyball

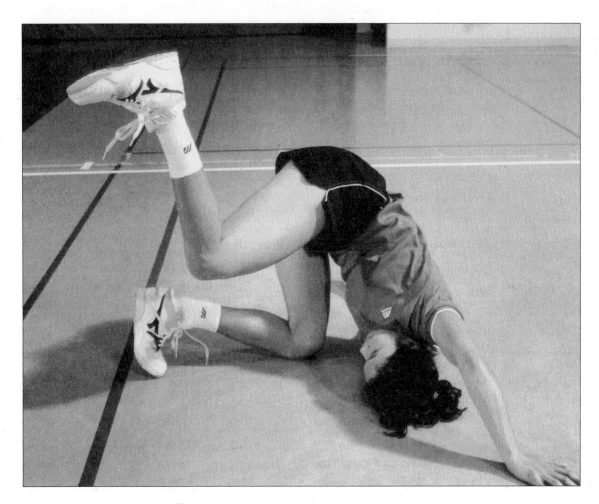

Outline

Proper execution is essential in playing winning volleyball. Fatigue, however, is a prime limiting factor to proper execution. How many times have you heard the statement, "I blew so many easy spikes," or "I cramped up"? These excuses can often be attributed to fatigue.

Injuries such as pulled muscles (strains), stretched ligaments (sprains), and muscle soreness are often the direct result of fatigue. As players get tired they make more physical errors, leading to injury. Being in shape for volleyball can help you avoid these pitfalls and increase your enjoyment from playing the game.

Increasing the Capacity of Your Cardiovascular System

Increasing the capacity of your cardiovascular system (heart, lungs, and arteries) is essential to supplying oxygen to all of your muscles for a period of time long enough to maintain the pace of an extended game or an all-day tournament.

Developing muscular endurance is also important. The muscles that are used continually during a match must have the ability to absorb oxygen and other fuels so that they do not tire. The legs (calf and thigh muscles) and the hitting arm (triceps, rotator cuff, and upper chest muscles) are most subject to fatigue, and must be exercised for endurance.

Strong muscles are a great help when that extra step, snap, rotation, jump, or support is needed. Specific strength-building exercises can also help prepare the body to withstand the strain of competition with less chance of injury. (See Chapter 16 for strength exercises.)

Flexibility is also desirable to enable you to perform quick body twists and the various volleyball skills without injuring your muscles.

The Overload Principle

The main factor in improving fitness of any kind is the overload principle. "Overload" means to push yourself each time to do a little more than you are accustomed to doing. Without this factor, there will be no improvement.

There are three ways to overload: intensity, duration, and frequency.

- *Intensity:* How hard you do something
- *Duration:* How long you do something
- *Frequency:* How often you do something

Intensity of exercise can be measured by monitoring your pulse rate, either during or immediately following exercise. The higher the pulse rate, the harder the heart is working. A task should become progressively easier as your condition improves, thus enabling you to work at higher intensities (such as all-out play for a longer period of time).

Intensity means playing at an elevated degree of speed, power, and concentration. All-out play—going full blast for every point and side out, pressing your opponent, and cutting down rest time between serves—puts pressure on your opponents.

Duration is measured by how long a period of time you continue to exercise—playing for longer periods of time each time you play, and gradually conditioning the heart to work a little longer without rest.

Frequency is measured by how often or how many times a week you play, run, or lift weights. Running four times per week instead of three times is an increase in frequency.

In order to improve the cardiovascular system, you must overload one or more of these principles of fitness; the safest and easiest on the body is frequency. You can overload on frequency by playing more times per week at the same intensity.

Aerobic Training

The cardiovascular system can be improved through the performance of exercises that elevate the pulse rate for an extended period of time. These activities, known as *aerobic exercises*, increase the body's ability to supply oxygen to its cells.

In order to contract (or shorten), muscle cells need fuel, which they receive from blood cells in the form of nutrients. The nutrients are metabolized from the food we eat. Oxygen is necessary for the cells to utilize these nutrients. When the heart and lungs cannot supply oxygen at a rate fast enough to keep up with the demands placed upon them by the body (a phenomenon known as oxygen debt), fatigue sets in and efficiency decreases.

Aerobic exercises train, or condition, the body to adapt to this demand by increasing the efficiency of the mechanisms involved—the heart, lungs, and arteries. They do this by forcing the heart to work much harder than normal for 20 to 30 minutes.

A *training effect* increases the efficiency of the lungs, allowing them to process more air with less effort; increases the efficiency of the heart, allowing it to pump more blood with each stroke; increases the number and size of the small blood vessels (capillaries); increases total blood volume; and improves the tone of your muscles and blood vessels.

The bottom line is that exercising aerobically increases maximal oxygen consumption by improving the efficiency of supply and delivery. You can select any activity that maintains your pulse in the target pulse zone (defined in the next section) for an extended period of time. The most commonly recommended activities are running, jogging, cycling, stationary running, rope jumping, walking, and swimming.

Aerobic activities are those that elevate the pulse rate to a level high enough to attain a training effect, but not so high as to cause fatigue or the need for a rest. The individual should be able to continue the exercise for a length of time long enough to attain a training effect.

Checklist of Benefits of the Aerobic Training Effect

1. *Increased efficiency of the lungs*—the lungs can process more air with less effort.
2. *Increased efficiency of the heart*—the stroke volume of the heart is increased, and the heart can pump more blood with each stroke.
3. *Increased number and size of blood vessels*—the arteries become more effective and capillaries increase in number.
4. *Increased total blood volume*—the body produces more blood cells to meet greater demands.
5. *Improved muscle tone*—the muscles become fitter and the muscle layer of the arteries becomes stronger.
6. *Fat weight changed to lean weight*—increase of lean body mass (percentage of muscle in the body).
7. *Increased maximal oxygen consumption*—the efficiency of the supply and delivery of oxygen to the cells is improved.

Target Pulse Rate

One way to ensure that you are exercising aerobically is to monitor your pulse rate to keep it in the *target pulse zone*, the pulse rate the body should maintain to reap the benefits of aerobic training. To determine your target pulse zone, first find your maximum exercise pulse, which is determined by subtracting your age from 220. Your target pulse zone is between 65 and 90 percent of your maximum exercise pulse. If the exercise is too intense, the pulse will rise above the upper limit of your target pulse zone and breathing will become more difficult as a result of your body's attempt to keep up with this extreme oxygen demand. For example, for a 20-year-old person,

220
−20 years old
‾‾‾‾‾‾
200 x 90% (.9) = 180
200 x 65% (.65) = 130

The target pulse zone is between 130 and 180.

A 20-year-old person should maintain a pulse rate of 130 to 180 for 20 to 30 minutes for the body to receive the benefits of aerobic training. This should be done a minimum of three or four times each week. (See the box for the more complicated Karvonen formula that is more generally used today.)

The key to being able to receive maximum benefits from aerobic activities is to exercise longer, not harder; low-intensity, long-lasting, continuous aerobic

The Karvonen Formula

The Finnish scientist M. J. Karvonen has improved on the simple formula of 220 minus your age as the maximum heart rate. He starts with that number, but then subtracts the resting pulse rate to determine the "heart rate reserve."

1. First take 220 minus your age ____. This is your maximum heart rate (MHR).

   Next, determine your resting heart rate while lying in bed in the morning before you get up. Use your index and middle fingers and locate your pulse, either on the side of your neck (carotid artery) or on the wrist just above the thumb. Count the number of pulse beats in a minute or take your pulse for 15 seconds and multiply by 4 to determine the total for a minute.

2. Resting heart rate (pulse rate) (rest HR) ____

3. Subtract your resting heart rate from the maximum pulse rate.

   MHR ____ − rest HR ____ = ____ heart rate reserve (HRR)

   Now you will determine your maximum and minimum pulse rates for an effective workout. For the average person, your high end will be your heart rate reserve multiplied by 80 percent (.80) added to your resting pulse rate.

4. ____ (HRR) × .80 = ____ + ____ (rest HR) = ____ maximum desirable heart rate during exercise

   Next find the minimal acceptable level for your workout by multiplying your heart rate reserve (HRR) by 60 percent (.60), added to your resting pulse rate.

5. ____ (HRR) × .60 = ____ + ____ (rest HR) = ____ minimal desirable heart rate during exercise

   These two percentages (60 and 80 percent) are not set in stone. If you have medical problems or are in very poor condition, you might use a number between 40 and 55 percent to set your minimal pulse rate. If you are very fit or a competitive athlete, you might use 85 or 90 percent to set your high-end exercise pulse rate.

   Here is an example of how a 20-year-old would determine her target training pulse range. Assume that her resting pulse rate is 70.

   Minimum target heart rate (220 − 20 = 200 − 70 = 130) × .60 = 78 + 70 = 148

   Maximum target heart rate (220 − 20 = 200 − 70 = 130) × .80 = 104 + 70 = 174

   For a 40-year-old with a resting pulse of 65, the target heart rates would be:

   Minimum target heart rate (220 − 40 = 180 − 65 = 115) × .60 = 69 + 65 = 134

   Maximum target heart rate (220 − 40 = 180 − 65 = 115) × .80 = 92 + 65 = 157

training periods help your body become able to continue performing for longer periods of time and to delay the onset of oxygen debt and fatigue while playing volleyball.

Anaerobic Training

Another type of exercise is that which demands oxygen at a faster rate than the body can provide—anaerobic exercises. Anaerobic literally means without oxygen. Anaerobic activities are so intense that they cannot be maintained for a long period of time. Exercises or sports involving stop-and-go activity, such as volleyball, tennis, and soccer usually require both aerobic and anaerobic conditioning because they have periods of intensity and times of inactivity. They are aerobic because the games last a long time, and they are anaerobic because of their start-and-stop nature.

Examples of anaerobic activities are running a 100-yard dash, weightlifting, or long, continuous rallies in volleyball. After engaging in such activities for a short time, the individual must stop and rest, usually breathing fast and deep to allow the body to replenish its oxygen stores. During anaerobic activities the pulse may be extremely elevated and breathing irregular (panting).

Volleyball often has periods of very intense activity so the body must be conditioned for these bursts of all-out activity. This conditioning can be attained in practice by playing more intensely for longer periods of time, resulting in an overload.

Other activities that may increase the body's ability to maintain a high intensity level are those that bring the pulse rate above the target pulse zone. Examples of this type of activities are running sprints, bicycle sprints, running up long flights of stairs, continuous jumping, and other explosive activities.

✓ *Checklist Comparing Aerobics and Anaerobics*

These two types of activities have contrasting characteristics, as shown below:

Characteristics

Aerobics	Anaerobics
Low intensity	High intensity
High duration	Low duration
Pulse slightly elevated	Pulse highly elevated
Continuous, uninterrupted workouts	Workouts interrupted by rests
Regular breathing	Irregular breathing; panting
No oxygen debt	Oxygen debt; fatigue
Burns fat and carbohydrates as fuel	Burns carbohydrates as primary fuel

Drills

Training is specific. The best way to get into shape for volleyball is to play and practice volleyball. Drills that require continual running and jumping are best for accomplishing this. A blocking drill with two spikers, one right and one left, forcing the blockers to block on one side of the court, then quickly moving to the other side and blocking, then returning, is an example of a drill that conditions the player anaerobically.

Summary

1. Conditioning can provide the means for a player to be able to maintain a high skill level throughout the entire game and avoid errors and injuries that may be attributed to fatigue.
2. Training is specific. In order to get into shape to play volleyball, you must play and practice volleyball.
3. Volleyball demands improvement of the cardiopulmonary system, strengthening of the muscles, and an increase in the flexibility of the joints.
4. For best results, the overload principle should provide the basis of your fitness program.
5. There are three ways to overload: intensity, duration, and frequency.
6. Aerobic training can improve the efficiency of the cardiovascular system.
7. Aerobic training results in the phenomenon known as the *training effect*.
8. Anaerobic exercises are activities of higher intensity and shorter duration, while aerobic exercises are activities of lower intensity and longer duration.
9. In order to benefit from the results of aerobic training, the pulse must remain in the target pulse zone all during the activity.
10. Since volleyball is primarily an anaerobic activity, improved fitness can be gained through playing volleyball at a more intense level for longer periods of time and by activities that duplicate these high-intensity demands, such as, sprinting, jumping, and other explosive activities.

16   *Strength and Flexibility*

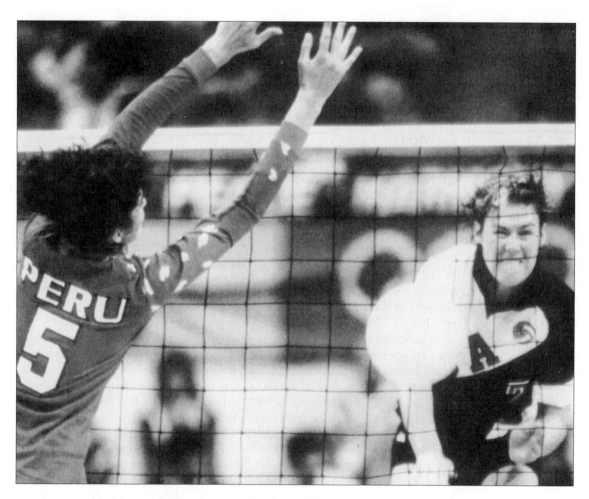

Outline

Volleyball players may not realize how much strength they need for the game. The jumping ability needed to spike or block a ball or the quickness required to dig a hit or a serve require both strength and flexibility.

It was only a few years ago that strength training for athletes was taboo. Now it is a necessity. The idea that working with weights makes people musclebound has given way to the knowledge that strength and flexibility training are essentials for every athlete.

Male athletes were the first to use resistance training. The shot putters and discus throwers led the way. Then it was the football players. Soon every athlete—male and female—found that strength training could greatly increase their abilities. As a volleyball player, you too can profit from strengthening your body.

Warming Up for Practice, Strength Workout, or Games

While traditionally it has been common to stretch prior to physical activity, recent research indicates that stretching before the workout is not always recommended. It may increase the risk of injury and reduce one's potential strength.

We know that we are all individuals with individual potentials or problems relative to our muscles and connective tissues. Some people like to do stretching exercises as part of their warm-up; others do not. It may help some people while hurting others. You may need to experiment with stretching versus not stretching in your warm-up. If you stretch, you may want to experiment with the types of stretches you do and whether you stretch to the maximum degree possible.

Research on stretching has not answered all—or even most—of our questions on whether or how to stretch. Is stretching a poor warm-up for a distance runner but a necessary factor for a high-jumper or dancer? We don't know. Distance runners are currently studied more often than other athletes in terms of the desirability of stretching. So far, the results indicate that for long-distance running, stretching may not be effective in preventing injuries.

A 1983 survey of 500 runners found that those who warmed up had more injuries than those who did not (87.7 percent vs. 66 percent) and the frequency of injuries increased with the length of the warm-up. It is assumed that stretching was part of the warm-up, but this was not specifically asked[1]. A few years later, a survey of 10K runners in the national championships found that those who stretched had more injuries. But it is not known whether those who stretched did so because they already had an injury and assumed that the stretching would protect them from further injury[2].

---

[1] J.A. Kerner and J.C. D'Amico, "A statistical analysis of a group of runners," *Journal of the American Podiatry Assn.* 73(3) 1983, pp. 160–164).

[2] S.J. Jacobs and B.L. Berson, "Injuries to runners: A study of entrants to a 10,000-meter race." *American Journal of Sports Medicine* 14(2) 1986, pp. 151–155.

Checklist for Workout Progression

1. Do a general body warm-up such as jogging, running in place while swinging your arms, or jumping jacks.
2. Practice your movements (such as a serve or spike) slowly at first so that your muscles warm up effectively.

In a study of recreational distance runners over a whole year it was found that those who sometimes stretched had more injuries than those who always stretched or those who never stretched. But those who never stretched had fewer new injuries than those who stretched[3]. While the above studies cast a doubt on the effectiveness of stretching for distance runners, certainly more and better research needs to be done.

In some activities you can stretch too long or too far in your warm-up. If you are entering a sprint race, on the track or in the pool, you would want your muscle fibers to be tighter and "stiffer." Too much stretch can slow you down. This is also true of jumpers—high jump or long jump—as well as swimmers and weightlifters. But if you are getting ready for a tennis match, a long run, or a leisurely afternoon of skiing, stretching should not be a problem[4].

For volleyball players we don't have hard evidence, but the indications are that stretching might reduce one's jumping and hitting abilities. More research is now being conducted into the effectiveness of warm-up stretching for various types of activities. The research indicates that your warm-up should allow for working up to maximum leg and arm force so that jumping and hitting can be done with full force.

General Strength Program

Every athlete should work on a general body-conditioning program before starting exercises designed for volleyball. A general body-strengthening program would include the following exercises:

- Bench press
- Triceps exercise (such as a triceps extension)
- Shoulder (military) press

---

[3] S.D. Walter, et al, "The Ontario cohort study of running-related injuries," *Archives of Internal Medicine* 149(11) 1989, pp. 2561–2564.

[4] G. Wilson, *Applied resistance training: A scientific approach*. Southern Cross University, NSW, Australia, 1998, Ch. 9, p. 25, unpublished manuscript.

- Biceps curl
- Squats
- Calf raises
- Hip abduction and adduction
- Lats
- Clean lifts
- Sit-ups
- Back arches

 Checklist for General Muscle Strength

1. Shoulder strength (bench press and shoulder press)
2. Arm strength (biceps curls and triceps extensions)
3. Leg strength (squats, calf rises)
4. Hip (abduction and adduction)
5. Upper back (lat exercises)
6. Lower back (back extensions)
7. Abdominals (curl-ups)
8. General body (cleans)

Specific Program for Volleyball

While an overall body building program may be good for everyone, there are specific exercises that can be particularly beneficial to athletes with special interests. Abdominal and lower-back strength are useful in nearly every sport. Volleyball players should strengthen their shoulders, arms, and wrists as well as their leg muscles.

How many repetitions and *how much weight* you use in the following exercises depends on your goals. For pure strength, you should be exhausted in one to three repetitions—but pure strength is not your only concern for volleyball. You want a certain amount of strength and you want muscular endurance, so you should do from 20 to over 50 repetitions. But any number of reps will help build strength and endurance.

Using a partner to provide "manual resistance" can actually be better than using weights. Your partner can adjust the pressure to make you work to a maximum level on each repetition. Weights can't do this; only partners and "isokinetic" machines have this capability. So if you are using a partner, don't imagine that you are not getting the best strength workout—in fact, that partner is probably entitled to a good dinner once a week for helping you to develop your "habit."

In the following outline of exercises for volleyball, several exercises are listed under each muscle group (such as front of deltoids, rotator cuff, or abdominals). You need choose only one of the options for your personal program.

Upper Shoulders

The shoulders are involved in every lifting, throwing, and hitting activity. They are therefore very important in volleyball competition. The front, top, and back of the shoulders are called the *deltoids*.

Front of deltoids

1. To exercise the front of the deltoids, while standing use two dumbbells. With a dumbbell in each hand and your palms pointed inward, raise the dumbbell as high as possible directly in front of you. The exercise can be done with both arms working at the same time or you can alternate them.

Top of deltoids

2. While standing with dumbbells in your hands and at your side, lift the dumbbells to the side and directly overhead with the backs of your hands staying on top of the dumbbells. (If you turn your hands palms up, you will be able to lift more weight because you will be allowing the upper chest muscles—your pectorals—to join in the work. You probably don't want this.)

Back of deltoids

3. While lying face down on a bench or standing while bending forward at a 90-degree angle at your waist, and with your head on a table or against a wall to reduce the pressure on the lower spinal disks, raise the dumbbells from directly below the shoulders sideways as far up as they will go. Keep your arms straight.

Rotator cuff

The rotator cuff muscles turn the upper arm in the shoulder socket. These very important muscles come into play in most throwing and hitting actions. They are particularly important in throwing a baseball and in spiking or serving a volleyball. Because these muscles are quite small, they are often injured. They should therefore be exercised for both maximum strength and for injury prevention.

4. While lying on your back on a bench or on the floor, holding a dumbbell with your elbow at a 90-degree angle to your side, bring the dumbbell to a vertical position, then continue the action until the weight is touching your abdomen. Return to the starting position. This exercise will work two different actions of the rotator cuff muscles.

5. While standing, bent at the waist, and with dumbbells in each hand, pull the weights back toward your waist and turn them to the inside.

6. While lying on your back with your upper arm at a 90-degree angle to your shoulder and your elbow flexed at 90 degrees, move a dumbbell over and back. This action comes close to the actual action of an overhand serve or an attacking hit.

7. Pulleys give you better resistance than the dumbbell exercise illustrated in exercise 2. Sitting on the floor with your left side to the lower pulley of a machine, your left elbow next to your hip, and your left hand on the handle, pull the handle across your body by rotating your upper arm and keeping the elbow bent. From the same position, take the handle in your right hand and pull the handle across your body. Change to sitting with your right side to the machine and work each exercise.

Abdominals

Most people are aware of how important it is to have abdominal strength. It helps to keep our abdomens tucked in for better posture. In fact the abdominals, along with the lower back, are the two most important areas for strength in our bodies.

In athletics the abdominals help to stabilize the pelvis, so they are essential in every action involving the hip joints—running, jumping, swimming, gymnastics, and the hip rotation in a volleyball spike or serve.

In order to attempt to isolate your abdominals, lie on your back and bend your knees as much as possible so that the muscles that flex the hip joint (bringing the thighs forward and upward) will not work as much. You should also keep your hips (your belt) on the mat when doing an abdominal exercise. Whenever your hips are pulled off the mat or bench, your hip flexors are working. This is particularly harmful for girls and women, who generally have an excessive curvature in their lower backs. This curvature places a higher pressure on the outside of the disks in the lumbar (lower back) region, and may cause problems as women grow older.

Some hip flexion exercises can increase the curvature of the spine because there are muscles deep inside the pelvis that attach from the lumbar vertebrae (lower back) to the thigh bone. As these muscles get stronger, they pull in on the lower spine and increase the curvature. This extreme lower-back curve (technically called "lordosis") is often seen in female gymnasts.

1. Abdominal curl-ups are done by lying on the floor or on a bench with your knees bent and your hands on your chest. Curl your shoulders forward until your hips are about to leave the floor. You will usually be able to touch your elbows to your thighs. If you do curl-ups on an inclined board with your head lower than your feet, you will increase the resistance you are lifting.

   Most people are looking for muscular endurance so that they can hold their abdominal muscles flat longer. If this is what you want, do lots of curl-ups. If you are working for strength, hold weight plates on your chest in order to increase resistance.

Checklist for Abdominal Exercises

1. Bend your knees so that your hip flexors cannot contract effectively.
2. If your hips leave the bench or incline board, your hip flexors are contracting.
3. Think of yourself as curling up rather than sitting up.

Some people aren't sufficiently strong to do this exercise correctly the first time. If this is true for you, do the exercise this way. Grab the back of your thighs with your hands and pull yourself up to the proper position. When this becomes easy, use only one hand on one thigh to help you curl up. Soon you will be able to do the exercise without using your hands to assist you. The exercise is easier with your hands on your hips and harder with your hands on your chest.

2. Side sit-ups are done to get additional strength in the muscles on the side of your abdominal area (the obliques). For this exercise you will have to have your feet held down, or you can hook your feet under a barbell. Lying on your side with your feet securely held down, lift your shoulders from the mat or bench. This exercise will not only work the abdominal oblique muscles but also the muscles on one side of your lower back and the rectus abdominis on the side to which you are bending.

Lower Back

Exercises for the lower back are probably the most important for the average person to do since lower-back injuries, especially muscle pulls, are so common. The problem is that these muscles don't show when we are in our shorts so we often overlook them.

The lower-back muscles are particularly important in volleyball because of the quick bending movements involved. And of course they are essential in maintaining good posture because they are the muscles that hold our chests up by lifting our rib cages. They pull the back of the rib cage down. This raises the front of the rib cage and our chests come up with our ribs.

1. Back arches can be done on the floor. Just lie face down and raise your shoulders and knees slightly off the floor. You do not want a big arch because hyperextending the backbone is not a safe exercise.

2. In a gym there may be a "Roman chair" available; if so, this exercise increases the resistance you can gain in your exercise. In a Roman chair you lay face down with your hips on the small saddle, hook your feet under a bar, bend forward at the waist about 30 degrees, then straighten your back, being careful not to hyperextend. If you want strength, just hold weight plates or a dumbbell behind your head. If you want muscular endurance, do as many reps as you can.

Hip Flexors

The hip flexors bring our thighs forward, so they are essential in any running or jumping activity. As previously mentioned, hip flexion exercises might be harmful for some people, especially women. However, many people need strength in the hip flexor muscles. Volleyball players, like anyone who runs fast, must have hip flexor strength.

For those who would be susceptible to an excessive lower-back curvature, special precautions should be taken. They should keep the connective tissue in their lower backs flexible by doing toe-touching exercises while sitting. They should also keep their abdominals strong to reduce the tendency of the front of the hips to drop forward. (This tendency would increase the curve of the lower spine.)

Hip flexors are exercised when the thigh is brought forward. This can be done several ways. You can do them hanging or standing. You can do them without weights, with a weighted boot, or with an ankle attachment to a pulley on a weight machine.

1. While hanging from a high bar with both hands, bring your legs forward with your knees bent. Touch your knees to your chest.
2. While hanging from the high bar, bring your legs forward without bending your knees.
3. Using the lower pulley of a weight machine, hook your ankle into a handle or use an ankle strap to secure your ankle to the pulley. Raise your leg straight forward.
4. While standing, with or without weight boots, brace yourself with your arms, lift one leg forward as high as it will go. Bring it up slowly.
5. Leg lifts are done from the supine position (on your back). Lift one or both legs from the floor to the vertical position. Your abdominals will contract isometrically in this, as in all other hip flexion exercises. Be careful not to arch your back.

Wrist Flexion (Front of Forearms)

The wrist flexors are used in any throwing or hitting motion. They put the curve on a curve ball and the fast in a fast ball, and they bring the hand through the ball on a spike or serve. Wrist strength is also essential in setting the ball.

1. Sit down while straddling a bench. With a barbell in your hands, your palms up, and the back of your forearms on the bench, let the weight hyperextend your wrist then flex your wrist forward. This exercise can also be done with a dumbbell, exercising one wrist, then the other.

    Some people use a weight attached by a rope to a handle. The exerciser raises the weight by rolling the handle using alternate wrist movements. This is not good for maximum strength gain, but it is useful for increasing muscle size or muscular endurance.

2. The tennis ball squeeze assists in developing wrist strength and also develops strength in the fingers. Find an old, soft tennis ball and squeeze it repeatedly.

Wrist Extension (Back of Forearms)

The wrist extensors are important in stabilizing the wrist in any backhand action in tennis, racquetball, or golf. In volleyball they hold the hands back while making the passing platform.

While sitting and straddling a bench (as in the previous exercise) and with your hands grasping the barbell (palms down), let the barbell flex your wrists then extend your wrists upward. This exercise will strengthen the back of your forearms. You will probably be able to use only about two-thirds of the weight as you used in the wrist flexion exercise.

Hip Abduction

Hip abduction means moving your leg sideways on a lateral plane. It uses the muscles on the outside of the hips. It is used by anyone who wants to move laterally while facing ahead. It is important in volleyball, a game that involves lateral movement to get into position to hit a shot or to block.

1. If you have an abduction machine, sit in the seat, hook your legs into the stirrups, and push both legs outward.
2. With a partner, lie on your back with your partner holding the outside of your feet or lower legs. Push your legs apart as far as they will go with your partner resisting.
3. On a machine, use the lower pulley. While standing sideways to the machine at the low pulley station, hook the foot that is farthest from the pulley into the handle (or use an ankle strap) and pull your leg away from the machine.

Hip Adduction

Hip adduction exercises strengthen the muscles on the inside of the leg (the groin area). These muscles are also used in moving laterally.

1. With an adduction machine, sit in the seat, put your feet in the stirrups, and with your legs apart, squeeze them together.
2. With a partner, while sitting and with your legs spread, have your partner grasp your ankles and give you resistance as you squeeze your legs together.
3. On a machine with a low pulley, stand away from the machine and sideways to it; hook the foot that is nearest the pulley in the handle, squeeze your leg in toward your body, pulling the handle away from the machine.

Upper Legs and Hips

1. The *front of the thigh* (quadriceps) is very important in running and jump-ing, so strength in these muscles is essential for attackers and blockers. If you are in a gym, use the quadriceps machine. If not, get a partner. Sit on a table and have your partner place both hands on your ankle and give you resistance while you straighten your leg. If you don't have a partner, you can use an exercise rubber band.

2. The *back of the thigh* (hamstrings) must be strong for running and jumping and to counterbalance the quadriceps. Gyms have special machines for the hamstrings. If you don't have access to a machine, get your trusty partner, lie face down on the floor or a table, and have your partner push against your ankle as you lift your lower leg from the floor. Keep your knee on the floor.

3. The *back of the hips* (gluteals) work with your quads in jumping. To strengthen your upper rear hips—the muscles that share a lot of your power work with your quads, lie on a table face down with your hips on the table but your thighs past the table and your toes touching the floor. You can use a partner to resist your upward movement if you want more strength, or you can do it alone if you want more endurance—just do many repetitions. Start with one toe touching the floor while the other leg is brought as high as possible, then alternate legs. This will look like an exag-gerated kicking action for a person swimming the crawl stroke.

4. *Hip and knee extensions* give you greater force potential from your hips and knees, and are the best jumping exercises. Gyms have squat racks, sleds, or other machines that allow you to extend your legs. However, you can easily do them at home. Do a three-quarters knee-bend (don't bend your knees over 90 degrees), or you can do half knee-bends. For twice the amount of resistance, do your knee-bends with only one leg. To do a half squat, hold a tabletop to steady yourself. Using only one leg, bend down 45 to 90 degrees, then return to a standing position. By doing it on only one leg, you get the same effect as doing it with two legs while holding a bar-bell equal to your own weight.

Lower Legs

1. *Calf muscles (gastrocnemius)* exercises are done by simply rising up on your toes then bringing your heels back to the ground. Repeat many times for endurance. If you want more strength for jumping, balance yourself by holding a table or chair, then do the exercise using only one leg at a time—the right leg until it is exhausted, then the left leg until it is exhausted.

2. The *muscles inside and outside of your lower leg* help keep your knees and ankles from twisting, so if they are strong, they can prevent injuries. The best way to work these muscles is to sit down, cross one leg over the other with your raised foot just past your other knee. Place one hand on the out-

side of the foot and move your foot outward as you resist with your hand. (The scientific name for this movement is "eversion.") Then put the other hand on the inside of the foot, near the ball of your foot, and resist as you bring your foot inward (inversion).

Flexibility Exercises

Flexibility is generally defined as the range of motion of a joint[5]. Every volleyball player, just like other athletes, needs a certain amount of flexibility. To increase flexibility, stretching exercises should be done very slowly, then hold the stretch (static stretch), or stretch while moving (ballistic or dynamic stretch), but stretching should never be done with jerky movements.The slow static stretch is generally recommended for most stretching workouts[6].

A few simple flexibility exercises should be done after every workout, practice, or game. These exercises stretch your connective tissues so that flexibility is increased. Following is the preferred order for stretching exercises:

1. *Shoulder rotation*. Stand erect with your arms extended out to your sides. Rotate them forward in circles with your hands making circles of 12 to 15 inches. Do this for 15 seconds, then rotate your arms backward for 15 seconds.

2. *Seated shoulder and chest stretch*. Sit with your legs together with the back of your legs flat on the floor and with your body erect. "Walk" your hands backward to a comfortable stretch position. Concentrate on keeping your upper body straight and emphasize stretching the tissue in the front of your shoulder. Hold this position for 30 seconds.

3. *Groin*. While seated on the floor, put the soles of your feet together and pull them toward your hips with your hands. With your back straight, try to press your knees to the floor. Do this for 30 seconds.

4. *Lower back and hamstrings*. While sitting on the floor, spread your legs outward as far as possible. While keeping your back and legs straight, with your toes pointed up, reach your hands as far as possible toward your right ankle. Do this for 30 seconds, then reach for your left ankle for 30 seconds.

5. *Gluteal stretch*. Sit on the floor with your legs together and the back of your legs touching the floor. Grab your right heel with your left hand, pass your right arm under your right calf, and lift your right foot toward the midsec-

---

[5] Coaches Roundtable, "Prevention of Athletic Injuries Through Strength Training and Conditioning," *National Strength & Conditioning Association Journal,* 5(2), 1983, pp. 14–19; and ibid, "Flexibility," *NSCA Journal,* 6(4) 1984, pp. 10–22.

[6] S.P. Sady, et al., "Flexibility Training: Ballistic, Static, or Proprioceptive Neuromuscular Facilitation?" *Archives of Physical Medicine Rehabilitation,* 63(6) June 1982, pp. 261–263.

tion of your body. Keep your left leg extended and your upper body erect, and do the exercise for 30 seconds. Then do the same exercise with your left leg.

6. *Trunk twist.* While sitting on the ground with your legs straight, bend your right leg and cross it over your left leg and put your right foot flat on the ground. Reach your left arm around your bent leg as if you were trying to touch your hip. Place your right arm behind you as you slowly twist your head and neck until you are looking over your right shoulder. Hold for 30 seconds, then do the exercise on the other side.

7. *Thigh and groin stretch.* From a standing position, step forward with your left leg. Lean forward over your left leg while keeping your left foot flat on the floor. Push down with your right leg until you feel a good stretch in your thigh and groin area. You can put your hands on the ground for balance. Stretch for 30 seconds, then do it with the other leg.

8. *Triceps stretch.* While standing, pull your right elbow behind your head until you feel the stretch. Hold for 30 seconds and then repeat with the other arm.

9. *Triceps stretch.* With your left hand, pull your right elbow across your chest. Hold for 30 seconds.

10. *Calf stretch.* Stand three to four feet from a wall. With your hands on the wall, lean into the wall while keeping your legs straight. You should feel the stretch in the back of the ankles and the lower legs. It can also be done without a wall by striding forward, bending the forward leg and keeping the rear leg straight.

Plyometrics

Serious volleyball players often want to increase their jumping abilities beyond that which strength training can accomplish. Much recent scientific evidence centers on the "stretch-shortening" cycle. This is the term given to the action of a muscle when it is stretched under pressure, then quickly shortened. This gives the muscle more power; that is, the stretching of the muscle makes it more ready to shorten with greater intensity.

One example is to run, landing on your toes, then quickly begin the next stride. Jumping from a bench to the ground and immediately jumping back up to a second bench is another, and hopping is still another. When your muscles stretch under a load, then immediately contract, that extra energy is available from two sources. More muscle fibers are required to "catch" the load as you land, then this greater number of fibers seems to be able to contract in the jump. Also, energy is stored in the tendons and other connective tissues and can be added to the increased force of propulsion when the muscle contracts.

Plyometric exercises are geared to teach your muscles to increase their power (strength plus speed) by using this "stretch-shortening" action in an exercise. This helps both speed and jumping ability. Other examples of such exercises are hopping, especially down stairs; jumping down from a box and up to another; and bounding running. Some trained athletes can jump from a four-foot-high box to the floor then rebound jump to another four-foot-high box. However, you should not begin plyometric exercises until your muscles are sufficiently strong.

Summary

1. Every athlete should perform a general body strength workout that includes exercises for shoulders, biceps, triceps, abdominals, upper back, lower back, hips, and legs.

2. Every athlete should develop the specific strength, flexibility, muscular endurance, and cardiovascular endurance necessary for his or her chosen sport.

3. The volleyball player should then perform the specific muscular actions that are specially designed to improve success in this sport.

4. The abdominal and lower back areas are extremely important areas for strength.

5. To reach maximum potential in volleyball, players should do specific exercises that strengthen the body areas most used.

6. Stretching is needed to allow a person to be able to move through a full range of motion.

7. Stretches should be held at least 15 seconds and are more effective if held 30 seconds.

8. Stretches should be done slowly and held at the maximum stretching position (static stretch).

17 Nutrition for Better Conditioning

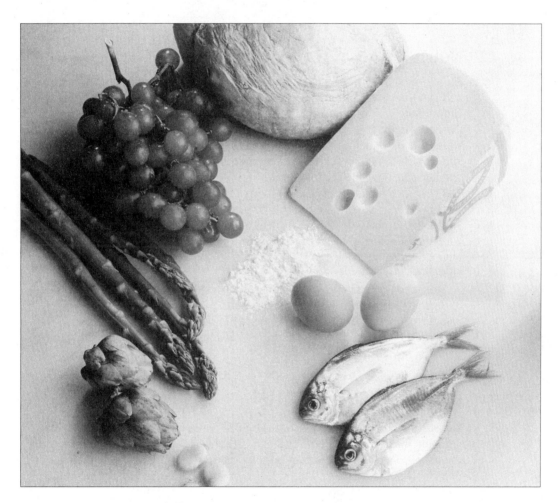

Outline

A long and full life requires exercise, an adequate diet, and play—both physical and mental, and a basic understanding of the science of nutrition is essential to healthy living. If you are going to play aggressive volleyball you will need adequate fuel for your athletic body. This chapter describes the basic elements of good nutrition. In the next chapter we will discuss how to apply these nutritional principles to your diet and weight management.

Nutrition

An informed person is aware of the nutrients necessary for minimal function, and can then put that knowledge into practice by developing a proper diet. Unfortunately, very few people consume even the minimum amounts of each of the necessary nutrients—protein, fat, carbohydrates, vitamins, minerals, and water (the essential nonnutrient). The first three nutrients listed (protein, fat, and carbohydrates) provide the energy required to keep us alive, in addition to making other specific contributions to our bodies.

The *calorie* measure used in counting food energy is really a kilocalorie—one thousand times larger than the calorie used as a measurement of heat in chemistry class. In one food calorie (kilocalorie), there is enough energy to heat one kilogram of water one degree Celsius, or to lift 3,000 pounds of weight one foot high. So those little calories you see listed on cookie packages pack a lot of energy.

Most people need about 10 calories per pound just to stay alive. If you plan to do something other than just lie in bed all day, you probably need about 17 calories per pound of body weight per day in order to keep yourself going. And if you decide to play a couple of hours of doubles at the beach, you can count on using a whole lot more calories.

Protein

Protein is made up of 22 *amino acids*, which consist of carbon, hydrogen, oxygen, and nitrogen. While both fats and carbohydrates contain the first three elements, nitrogen is found only in protein. Protein is essential for building nearly every part of the body—the brain, heart, organs, skin, muscles, and even the blood.

There are four calories in one gram of protein. Adults require 0.75 grams of protein per kilogram of body weight per day; this translates into one-third a gram of protein per pound. So an easy way to estimate your protein requirements in grams per day is to divide your body weight by three. For instance, if you weigh 150 pounds, you need about 50 grams of protein per day.

Physically active adults have been thought to require more protein than is recommended by the United States Recommended Daily Allowance (USRDA), which is set at .8 grams per kilogram of body weight per day. In fact, most active people do not need to eat additional protein if 12 to 15 percent of their total calories is protein. Since active individuals need to consume more calories per day than their inactive counterparts due to their increased energy expenditure, active adults who keep their protein intake at around 15 percent of their total calories will eat more protein per day and thereby fulfill their body's protein requirement. Excess protein consumption (above the body's requirement) is broken down and the calories are either burned off or stored as fat.

However, when you are involved in a strenuous strength training regimen, as you might be if you play competitive volleyball, it may be necessary to increase your protein intake percentage, depending on the number of total calories you consume per day.

In order for your body to make any kind of tissue, including muscle, you must first have all of the necessary amino acids. Your body can manufacture some of them, while you must get others from your food. Those amino acids that you must get from your food are called the *essential amino acids*, while the others that you can make are known as the *nonessential amino acids*. During childhood, nine of the 22 amino acids are essential, while in adulthood we acquire the ability to synthesize one additional amino acid, leaving us with eight essential amino acids.

Amino acids cannot be stored in the body, so we need to consume our minimum amounts of protein every day. If adequate protein is not consumed, the body immediately begins to break down tissue (usually beginning with muscle tissue) to release the essential amino acids. If even one essential amino acid is lacking, the other essential ones are not able to work to their capacities. For example, if methionine (the most commonly lacking amino acid) is present at 60 percent of the minimum requirement, the other seven essential amino acids are limited to near 60 percent of their potential. When they are not used, amino acids are excreted in the urine.

Animal products (fish, poultry, and beef) and animal byproducts (milk, eggs, and cheese) are rich in readily usable protein. This means that when you eat animal products or byproducts, the protein you consume can be converted into protein in your body because these sources have all of the essential amino acids in them. These foods are called *complete protein sources*.

Incomplete protein sources are any other food sources that provide protein but not all of the essential amino acids. Examples of incomplete proteins include peas and nuts. These food sources must be combined with other food sources that have the missing essential amino acids so that you can make protein in your body. Examples of complementary food combinations are rice and beans or peanut butter on whole wheat bread.

Another reason to be aware of complementary food combinations is that they enhance the absorption of the protein consumed. The person who is aware of the varying qualities of proteins can combine them to take advantage of the strengths of each. For example, if you eat flour at breakfast in the form of a piece of toast or coffeecake and wash it down with coffee, then drank a glass of milk at lunch, each of the protein sources would be absorbed by your body at a lower level. But if you ate bread with the milk at either meal, the higher protein values of both would be absorbed by your body immediately.

Fats

Fat is made of carbon, hydrogen, and oxygen. There are nine calories in a gram of fat. In the body, fat is used to develop the myelin sheath that surrounds the nerves. It also aids in the absorption of vitamins A, D, E, and K, which are the fat-soluble vitamins. It serves as a protective layer around our vital organs, and it is a great insulator against the cold. It is also a great concentrated energy source. And of course its most redeeming quality is that it adds flavor and juiciness to food!

Just as protein is broken down into different kinds of nitrogen compounds called amino acids, there are also different kinds of fats. There are three major kinds of fats, or fatty acids: saturated fats, monounsaturated fats, and polyunsaturated fats.

Saturated fats are "saturated" with hydrogen atoms. They are generally solid at room temperature and are most often found in animal fats, eggs, and whole milk products. Since these are the fats that are primarily responsible for raising the blood cholesterol level and hardening the arteries, they should be minimized in your diet.

Monounsaturated fats (oleic fatty acids) have room for two hydrogen ions to double-bond to one carbon. They are liquid at room temperature and are found in great amounts in olive, peanut, and canola (rapeseed) oils. Dietary monounsaturated fats have been shown to help the body excrete dietary cholesterol, thereby helping to prevent atherosclerosis, one type of arteriosclerosis.

Polyunsaturated fats (linoleic fatty acids) have at least two carbon double-bonds available, which translates into space for at least four hydrogen ions. Polyunsaturated fats are also liquid at room temperature and are found in the highest proportions in vegetable sources. Safflower, corn, and linseed oils are good sources of this type of fat. Polyunsaturated fatty acids of the omega-3 type may also contribute to the prevention of atherosclerosis.

We eat too much fat. The minimum requirement for fat in the diet is considered to be somewhere between 10 and 20 percent of the total calories consumed. The absolute maximum should be 30 percent, which is the amount now recommended for the American diet. While we as a society are still above this 30 percent value, we have been declining since the 1970s, and we need to keep that trend going. Most of us consume between 35 and 50 percent of our total calories in fats, with a very high percentage in saturated fats—the fats that we want to avoid.

Our high fat intake, most of which is saturated, tends to raise blood cholesterol levels in many people. If you are interested in decreasing the chances of developing hardened arteries by lowering your blood cholesterol level, it is recommended that you follow a diet low in fat (with the saturated fat intake at 10 percent or less of your total diet) and consume less than 300 milligrams of cholesterol daily. Or to put it another way, keep the total calories from fat under a third of your total intake and eat at least twice as much polyunsaturated and monounsaturated fats as saturated fats.

In the past, companies were allowed to identify the oil in a product on their labels as simply vegetable oil; under the Food and Drug Administration requirements made in 1976, they are now required to note whether it is corn oil, cottonseed oil, soybean oil, and so on, because some oils, even though they are not of animal origin, are very high in saturated fat. Palm kernel oil and coconut oil, often referred to as "tropical oils," are particularly high in saturated fats.

When you buy foods, especially cookies and crackers, always check the type of fat used. Avoid those with palm kernel oil and coconut oil. Also be aware of the hydrogenated oils used. While a hydrogenated safflower or canola oil may still have an acceptable fat ratio, a hydrogenated peanut or cottonseed oil may not contain the desired levels of unsaturated fats. Partially hydrogenated vegetable oils may contribute to the development of heart disease. The dietary use of hydrogenated corn oil stick margarine has been shown to increase LDL cholesterol levels when compared to the use of similar amounts of corn oil, also indicating an increased risk of heart disease.

In terms of controlling one's blood cholesterol level, dietary cholesterol is not as important as saturated fats in your diet. For this reason, saturated fats such as red meats, butter, egg yolks, chicken skin, and other animal fats should be greatly decreased. As an informed consumer, you may want to keep track of both your total fat intake and your intake of saturated fat to become better aware of your potential risk for heart disease. For example, one egg contains 5.6 grams of fat and only 0.7 grams of polyunsaturated fat, while an equal weight of hamburger contains 8.7 grams of fat and only 0.4 grams of polyunsaturated fats.

Carbohydrates

Carbohydrates are made from carbon, hydrogen, and oxygen, just as are fats, but "carbs" are generally a simpler type of molecule. There are four calories in a gram of carbohydrate. If carbohydrates are not utilized immediately for energy as sugar (glucose), they are either stored in the body as glycogen (the stored form of glucose) or synthesized into fat and stored. Some carbohydrates cannot be broken down by the body's digestive processes; these are called fibers and will be discussed later. Digestible carbohydrates can be separated into two categories: simple and complex. *Simple carbohydrates* are the most readily usable energy source in the body and include such things as sugar, honey, and fruit. *Complex carbohydrates* are the starches, which also break down into sugar for energy, but their breakdown is slower than with simple "carbs." Complex carbohydrates also bring with them various vitamins and minerals.

People in the United States often eat too many simple carbohydrates. These are often referred to as "empty calories," because they have no vitamins, minerals, or fibers. While a person who uses a great deal of energy can consume these empty calories without potential weight gain, most of us find these empty calories settling on our hips. The average person consumes 125 pounds of sugar per year, which is equivalent to one teaspoon every 40 minutes, night and day. Since each teaspoon of sugar contains 17 calories, this amounts to 231,000 calories or 66 pounds of potential body fat if this energy is not used as fuel for daily living.

High-carbohydrate diets that are especially high in sugar may be hazardous to one's health. They can increase the amount of triglycerides produced in the liver. These triglycerides are blood fats and are possible developers of hardened arteries. Also, a diet high in simple carbohydrates can lead to obesity, which can then result in the development of late-onset diabetes.

Fiber

Fiber is that part of the foods we take in that is not digestible. Fiber helps to move food through the intestines by increasing their peristaltic action. Vegetable fibers are made up chiefly of cellulose, an indigestible carbohydrate that is the main ingredient in the cell walls of plants. Plant-eating animals, such as cows, can digest cellulose. Meat-eating animals, such as humans, do not have the proper enzymes in their digestive tracts to metabolize cellulose.

Bran—the husks of wheat, oats, rice, rye, and corn—is another type of fiber. Bran is indigestible because of the silica in the outer husks. Some fibers, such as wheat bran, are also insoluble. The major function of fiber is to add bulk to the feces and to speed digested foods through the intestines. This reduces one's risk of constipation, intestinal cancer, appendicitis, and diverticulosis.

Some types of fibers are soluble; that is, they can absorb and eliminate certain substances such as dietary cholesterol. Pectin, commonly found in raw fruits (especially apple skins), oat and rice brans, and some gums from the seeds and stems of tropical plants (such as guar and xanthin) are examples of soluble fibers that pick up cholesterols as they move through the intestines.

Foods high in fiber are also valuable in weight-reducing diets because when foods pass more quickly through the digestive tract, the time available for absorption is reduced. Fiber also cuts the amount of hunger experienced by a dieter because it fills the stomach. A large salad with a diet dressing might give you very few calories, but it contains enough cellulose to fill your stomach, cut hunger, and move other foods through the intestinal passage.

Food processing often removes natural fiber from our food, and this is one of the primary reasons that we in the western world have relatively low amounts of fiber in our diet. For instance, white bread has only a trace of fiber—about nine grams in a loaf—while old-fashioned whole wheat bread has 70 grams. And when you peel a carrot or an apple, you remove much of the fiber.

Dietitians urge us to include more fiber in our diets. People should be particularly conscious of the benefits of whole-grain cereals, bran, and fibrous vegetables. Root vegetables (carrots, beets, and turnips) and leafy vegetables are very good sources of fiber. The average American diet has between 10 and 20 grams of fiber in it per day. This low level of fiber is believed to account for the fact that we have about twice the rate of colon cancer as do other countries

Checklist for Effective Eating

1. Eat 12 to 15 percent of your diet in proteins, preferably fish, fowl without skin, and beans.
2. Keep your fat intake between 10 and 30 percent of your total calorie intake, with saturated fat intake 10 percent or less and a higher proportion of monounsaturated fat.
3. Most of your diet should be complex carbohydrates (less-refined products) such as whole wheat, fruits, and vegetables.
4. It is recommended that people supplement with antioxidant vitamins (beta carotene, vitamins C and E).

whose citizens eat more fiber. This is why the National Cancer Institute has recommended that we consume between 25 and 35 grams of fiber per day.

Vitamins

Vitamins are organic compounds that are essential in small amounts for the growth and development of animals and humans. They act as enzymes (catalysts) that facilitate many of the body's processes to occur. Although there is controversy about the effects of consuming excess vitamins, nutritionists agree that we need a minimum amount of vitamins for proper functioning.

Some vitamins are soluble only in water; others need fat to be absorbed by the body. The water-soluble vitamins, B complex and C, are more fragile than the fat-soluble vitamins, because they are more easily destroyed by the heat of cooking, and if they are boiled, they lose some of their potency into the water. Since they are not stored by the body, they should be included in the daily diet. However, even though they are not stored in the body, it is still possible to ingest too many of some water-soluble vitamins. An excess demand may be placed on the kidneys for processing.

The fat-soluble vitamins, A, D, E, and K, need oils in the intestines to be absorbed by the body. They are more stable than the water-soluble vitamins and are not destroyed by normal cooking methods. Because they are stored in the body, there is the possibility of ingesting too much of them—especially vitamins A and D.

Although nutritional researchers disagree about whether vitamin supplements are necessary, many of them see the necessity for supplementation with the vitamins that neutralize free oxygen radicals. *Free oxygen radicals* are harmful substances produced by many natural body processes, air pollution, and smoke, and seem to be responsible for some cancers and other diseases. Physical exercise, for all of its benefits, is one producer of free oxygen radicals.

Supplementation with antioxidants (beta carotene, vitamins C and E) reduces free oxygen radicals in the body. Dr. Ken Cooper, the man who coined the term "aerobics" and developed the first world-recognized fitness program, suggests a minimum supplementation of 400 IU of vitamin E, 1,000 mg of vitamin C, and 25,000 units of beta carotene daily to counteract the potential damage done to the body by free oxygen radicals.

Minerals

Minerals are usually structural components of the body, but they sometimes participate in certain body processes. The body uses many minerals: phosphorus, calcium, and magnesium for strong teeth and bones; zinc for growth; chromium for carbohydrate metabolism; and copper and iron for hemoglobin production in the blood.

Iron is used primarily in developing hemoglobin, which carries oxygen in red blood cells. Women need more iron (18 milligrams a day) than men until they go through menopause, at which time their iron requirements drop to that of men (10 milligrams a day). Iron deficiency, common in women athletes, may impair athletic performance and should be corrected with supplementation.

Magnesium is the eighth most abundant element on the earth's surface. It seems to help activate enzymes essential to energy transfer. It is crucial for effective contraction of the muscles. Exercise depletes this element, so supplementation may be called for. When it is not present in sufficient amounts, twitching, tremors, and undue anxiety may develop.

Calcium is primarily responsible for building strong bones and teeth. For this reason, it seems obvious that a diet that is chronically low in calcium would have a negative effect on one's bone strength. Low calcium intake results in brittle and porous bones as one gets older, a condition known as osteoporosis. This is diagnosed when bone density shows a loss of 40 percent of the necessary calcium. It happens quite often in older people, especially women who have gone through menopause or have had their ovaries removed, because estrogen seems to protect against bone loss.

In teenage and young adult years, the inclusion of adequate calcium (which may be higher than the current Recommended Daily Allowance, or RDA) can aid in the development of peak bone mass, which can help prevent osteoporosis later on in life. Another contributing factor to osteoporosis is the imbalance of phosphorus to calcium in the typical diet. Calcium and phosphorous work together, and should be consumed on a one-to-one ratio. However, the average diet is much higher in phosphorus than calcium, leading to a leeching of calcium from the bones to make up for this imbalance.

Calcium is also necessary for strong teeth, nerve transmissions, blood clotting, and muscle contractions. Without enough calcium, muscle cramps often result. Skipping milk with its necessary calcium may be the cause of menstrual cramping for some girls. The uterus is a muscle, and muscles need both sodium and calcium for proper contractile functioning.

Phytochemicals

Phytochemicals (*phyto* is the Greek word for "plant") include thousands of chemical compounds that are found in plants. Some of these are vitamins, and while many have no known effect on us, more and more are being found to be highly beneficial.

In the past, the phytonutrients found in fruits and vegetables were classified as vitamins: Flavonoids were known as vitamin P, cabbage factors (glucosinolates and indoles) were called vitamin U, and ubiquinone was vitamin Q. Tocopherol somehow stayed on the list as vitamin E. Vitamin designation was dropped for other nutrients because specific deficiency symptoms could not be established. "Vita" means "life," so if the compound could not be found to be absolutely essential for life, it was dropped as a "vitamin," but is now classified as a phytochemical.

Various phytochemicals have been found to reduce the chance of cancers developing, reduce the chance of heart attack, reduce blood pressure, and increase immunity factors. Few of these have been reduced to pill form like vitamin pills, so they must be consumed in fruits and vegetables daily. It is suggested that each of us consume at least five servings of raw fruits or vegetables daily. Since many phytochemicals are heat sensitive, cooking can destroy some or all of the active ingredients.

We are a long way from developing highly effective phytochemical supplements, because there are so many elements and they may be destroyed in the processing. Garlic pills, for example, are available. However, in the deodorized versions, some active ingredients have been removed—they were in the chemicals that give garlic its "aroma."

Several types of phytochemicals are being studied. *Plant sterols* are somewhat similar to the animal sterol cholesterol but are unsaturated. These plant sterols compete for the same sites and thereby lower the blood cholesterol levels by as much as 10 percent. Soy is a good source for such sterols. Most green and yellow vegetables, and particularly their seeds, contain essential sterols.

Phenols have the ability to block specific enzymes that cause inflammation. They also modify the prostaglandin pathways and thereby protect blood platelets from clumping, thereby reducing the risk of blood clots. Blue, blue-red, and violet colorations seen in berries, grapes, and purple eggplant are due to their phenolic content.

Flavonoids is the name for a large group of compounds found primarily in tea, citrus fruits, onions, soy, and wine. Some can be irritating, but others seem to reduce heart attack risk. For example, the phenolic substances in red wine inhibit oxidation of human LDL cholesterol. The biologic activities of flavonoids include action against allergies, inflammation, free radicals, liver toxins, blood clotting, ulcers, viruses, and tumors.

Terpenes such as those found in green foods, soy products, and grains comprise one of the largest classes of phytonutrients. The most intensely studied terpenes are carotenoids—as evidenced by the many recent studies on beta carotene. Only a few of the carotenoids have the antioxidant properties of beta carotene. These substances are found in bright yellow, orange, and red plant pigments found in vegetables such as tomatoes, parsley, oranges, pink grapefruit, and spinach.

Limonoids are a subclass of terpenes found in citrus fruit peels. They appear to protect lung tissue and aid in detoxifying harmful chemicals in the liver.

Recent research confirms suspicion of the effects of soy products and related foods, which have long been used in Asian diets. It has long been observed that Asian women do not experience the problems of menopause, such as hot flashes, that western women commonly endure, but until recently, no theories have been advanced. Now we realize that a major factor is the fact that the Asians eat more vegetables, particularly soybeans.

It is phytoestrogens—plant chemicals that mimic the effects of the female hormone estrogen—that seem to be the major factor. These plant-like estrogens have similar effects to the natural estrogen in reducing heart disease, maintaining brain functions, reducing the incidence of breast cancer, and reducing softening of the bones (osteoporosis). In addition, other positive effects, which may or may not be related to estrogen intake, also occur, such as reduction in cancers (prostate, endometrial, bowel) and the effects of alcohol abuse[1].

Water

Water is called the essential nonnutrient because it has no nutritional value, yet without it we would die. Water makes up approximately 60 percent of the adult body, while an infant's body is nearly 80 percent water. Water cools the body through perspiration, carries nutrients to and waste products from the cells, helps cushion our vital organs, and is an essential element of all body fluids.

The body has about 18 square feet of skin that contains about 2 million sweat glands. On a comfortable day, a person perspires about a half-pint of water. Somebody exercising on a severely hot day may lose as much as seven quarts of water. If this is not replaced, severe dehydration can result. It is therefore generally recommended that we daily drink eight 8-ounce glasses of water or the equivalent in other fluids. This amount is dependent on the climate in which you live, the altitude at which you live, the type of foods that you eat, and the amount of activity that you participate in on a day-to-day basis. Volleyball can be very strenuous and makes us sweat—so be sure to drink plenty of water before and during practice or games.

---

[1] S.A. Bingham et al, "Phyto-oestrogens: Where are we now?" *British Journal of Nutrition*, May 1998, 79(5) 393–406; S. T. Willard and L. S. Frawley, "Phytoestrogens have agonistic and combinatorial effects on estrogen-responsive gene expression in MCF-7 human breast cancer cells," *Endocrinology*, April 1998, 8(2), 117–121; T. B. Clarkson, "The potential of soybean phytoestrogens for postmenopausal hormone replacement therapy," *Proceedings of the Society of Experimental Biological Medicine*, March 1998, 217(3), 365–368.

Summary

1. The basic macronutrients are protein, fats, and carbohydrates.

2. Proteins are made of amino acids. Eight of these are considered to be essential and should be consumed daily.

3. Our bodies need fats, but they should be limited to 10 to 30 percent of our daily calorie intake.

4. Saturated fats and cholesterol are risk factors for heart disease.

5. The greatest percentage of our diets should be in complex carbohydrates, which contain vitamins, minerals, and fiber.

6. While proteins, fats, and carbohydrates (macronutrients) provide most of the nutrients we consume, the micronutrients—vitamins, minerals, and phytochemicals—are also essential.

7. Vitamins break down macronutrients and accomplish other essential body functions.

8. Free oxygen radicals are harmful byproducts of living that can be reduced by some vitamins (beta carotene, vitamins C and E).

9. Minerals are necessary building blocks of the body and are essential in all tissue.

10. Phytochemicals are desirable—and possibly necessary—elements found in plants, and may aid us in obtaining a higher level of nutrition.

11. Vitamin supplementation may be necessary for many people; most of us apparently profit from antioxidant supplementation.

12. Water is essential to all the body's functions; eight glasses of water a day is recommended.

18 Sensible Eating and Weight Management

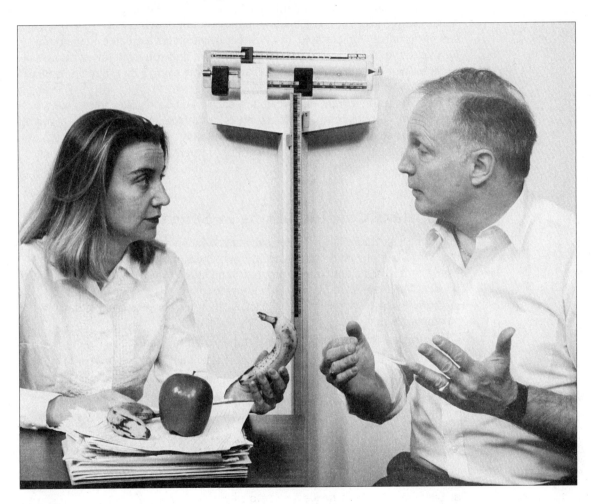

Outline

To eat sensibly, you must understand the basic principles of nutrition discussed in Chapter 17. Necessary nutrients must occur in your diet in proper quantities, and the calories you consume must be the amount necessary in order to maintain your desired weight. If you don't maintain your optimal weight, you may develop obesity and the diseases associated with obesity, such as diabetes, high blood pressure, and heart disease.

There are other factors that the sensible eater must understand. Caloric needs change according to climate and the amount of activity in which the person participates. For example, hot weather necessitates a greater intake of fluids due to the loss of water through perspiration, and you need fewer calories because your body does not need to burn as many calories to maintain its 98.6° Fahrenheit temperature.

A person using a great many calories, such as a beach volleyball player, needs more carbohydrates, but it is a myth that athletes need a great deal more protein than non-athletes. While caloric needs may nearly double for the athlete who is expending a great deal of energy, protein needs are increased only slightly—usually less than 30 percent.

Important Considerations in Selecting Your Diet

The U.S. Department of Agriculture has devised a suggested diet guide called the Food Guide Pyramid. Its base is grain products, next comes fruits and vegetables, then meats and animal products, and at the top some fats or sweets if needed. There are six food groups in the pyramid:

- Grain products (breads, cereals, pastas): six to eleven servings per day recommended
- Vegetables: three to five servings per day recommended
- Fruits: two to four servings per day recommended
- High-protein meats and meat substitutes (meat, poultry, fish, beans, nuts, tofu/soy, eggs): two to three servings per day recommended
- Milk products: two servings per day for adults, three for children recommended
- Extra calories, if needed, from fats and/or sweets

Grain products provide the carbohydrates needed for quick energy. A serving size is one slice of bread, an ounce of dry cereal, or a half-cup of cooked cereal, pasta, or rice. Daily needs are six to eleven servings.

Grains are rich in B vitamins, some minerals, and fiber. Whole grains are the best sources of fibers. Refining grains or polishing rice reduces the fiber, the mineral content, and the B vitamins. This occurs in white and wheat bread (not whole wheat), pastas, pastries, and white rice. Flour is often refortified with three of the B complex vitamins, but seldom with the other essential nutrients.

If you want to reduce your cholesterol level, thereby reducing your chances of heart disease, reduce your chances of developing gallstones, or have a softer bowel movement, eat more of the soluble fibers (oat bran cereals, whole grain

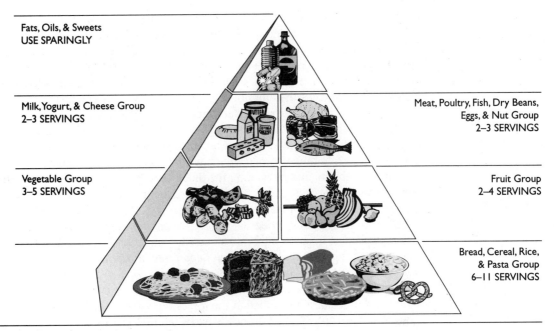

Fats, Oils, & Sweets
USE SPARINGLY

Milk, Yogurt, & Cheese Group
2–3 SERVINGS

Meat, Poultry, Fish, Dry Beans,
Eggs, & Nut Group
2–3 SERVINGS

Vegetable Group
3–5 SERVINGS

Fruit Group
2–4 SERVINGS

Bread, Cereal, Rice,
& Pasta Group
6–11 SERVINGS

The Food Guide Pyramid

bread with oats, rice bran, carrots, potatoes, apples, and citrus juices that contain pulp). If your concern is reducing your risk of intestinal cancers, appendicitis, and diverticulosis, eat more of the insoluble fibers (whole wheat breads and cereals, corn cereals, prunes, beans, peas, nuts, most vegetables, and polished rice).

Vegetables are rich in fibers, beta carotene, some vitamins and minerals. Among the most nutritious vegetables are broccoli, carrots, peas, peppers, and sweet potatoes. If you are trying to lose weight, many vegetables are high in water and in fibers but low in calories. Among these are all greens (lettuce, cabbage, celery) as well as cauliflower. Actually, most vegetables are quite low in calories. You need three to five servings daily; a serving size is a half-cup of raw or cooked vegetables or a cup of raw leafy vegetables.

Fruits are generally high in vitamin C and fiber, and they are also relatively low in calories. You should have two to four servings daily; a serving size is one-fourth cup of dried fruit, a half-cup of cooked fruit, three-quarters cup of fruit juice, a whole piece of fruit, or a wedge of a melon.

Protein sources such as meats, egg whites, nuts, and beans are also high in minerals and vitamins B6 and B12. You need two to three servings a day; a serving is two and one-half ounces of cooked meat, poultry or fish, two egg whites, four tablespoons of peanut butter, one and one-fourth cups of cooked beans. A McDonald's "Quarter-Pounder" would give you two servings. The hidden eggs in cakes and cookies also count. The best meat products to eat are fish, egg whites, and poultry without the skin.

Red meat not only has a relatively low quality of protein (ranked after egg white, milk, fish, poultry, and organ meats), but it is linked to both cancers (two and a half times the risk for colon cancer) and heart disease. It also carries a great amount of fat, even if the fat on the outside is trimmed off. There is also a lot of cholesterol in the meat and fat of all land animals. Taking the skin off poultry greatly reduces the amount of fat and cholesterol that will be consumed, because poultry carry much of their fat next to the skin.

Of the animal proteins, fish has a higher quality of protein than meat or poultry. Also, fish are able to convert polyunsaturated linolenic fatty acids from plants they eat into omega 3 oils, which work to prevent heart disease by reducing cholesterol and by making the blood less likely to clot in the arteries. They do this by interfering with the body's production of the prostaglandin thromboxane, which increases blood clotting.

Milk and milk products (cheeses, yogurt, ice cream) are high in calcium and protein as well as in some minerals (potassium and zinc) and riboflavin. Adults need two servings daily, while children need three; a serving is one cup of milk or yogurt, one and one-half ounces of cheese, two cups of cottage cheese, one and one-half cups of ice cream, or one cup of pudding or custard.

Fats and sweets are positioned at the top of the pyramid of foods. They should be eaten only if a person needs extra calories. Consuming more fat than the recommended maximum of 30 percent of one's diet can be quite harmful—particularly in causing cancers and hardened arteries. Most researchers suggest a maximum of 10 to 20 percent of the diet in fats, with most in the form of monounsaturated and polyunsaturated fatty acids.

Sweets may assist in the development of tooth caries (cavities), but are not otherwise harmful if calories are not a problem for you. An athlete consuming 5,000 calories in a day can probably eat candy bars and ice cream, but the person attempting to control their weight should avoid them.

In addition to merely consuming the right proportions of foods, a concerned person would implement several other precautions:

- Avoid milk fat by drinking nonfat milk and milk products; eating ice milk (3 percent fat) or frozen desserts made without milk fat; and eating no-fat or low-fat cheeses. Half of the calories in whole milk come from the 3 1/2 percent of the milk that is fat. Low-fat milk is reduced in fat calories by 40 percent. When low-fat milk is advertised as 98 percent fat-free, it is not that much better than whole milk, which is 96 1/2 percent fat-free. The fats in milk are highly saturated—the worst kind of fat—yet the protein quality of milk is second only to egg whites.

- Avoid egg yolks because they contain a great deal of cholesterol and saturated fat. They are second only to caviar (fish eggs) in cholesterol content. Egg whites, on the other hand, have the highest rating for protein quality and are one of the best things you can eat.

- Reduce salt, because it is related to high blood pressure; and sugars, because they give "empty" calories—calories without other nutrients such as vitamins or fiber.

- Reduce fats to between 10 and 20 percent of your total calories. Normal salad dressings contain about 70 calories per tablespoon. If calories are a problem, use fat-free dressing or vinegar or lemon juice only. Rather than a butter or margarine, buy a good tasty whole-grain bread and eat it without grease. If you must use grease, use olive oil, or perhaps olive oil and balsamic vinegar as they serve in many Italian restaurants. If calories are not a concern and you like sweets, use jelly or jam.

- Never fry foods in oil; use a non-stick pan. If you must have an oil, use canola (rapeseed), olive, or safflower oil. Stay away from all fried foods, including potato chips. Fried foods not only add calories and saturated fats, but they also increase one's chances for intestinal cancers—as do all fats.

Beverages

Beverages make up a large part of our diet. We often don't think too much about the kinds of liquids we drink. The most nutritious drinks have been rated by the Center for Science in the Public Interest according to the amount of fat and sugar (higher content = lower rating), and their amount of protein, vitamins, and minerals (higher content = higher rating). Here are some sample results: skim or nonfat milk was rated +47, whole milk +38 (the lower rating was because of its fat content), orange juice +33, Hi-C +4, coffee 0, coffee with cream –1, coffee with sugar –12, Kool-Aid –55, and soft drinks –92.

Milk is the best beverage for most people. Children should have three to four cups each day, while adults should drink two cups. Our need for milk can be satisfied by other dairy products. For example, two cups of milk are equivalent to three cups of cottage cheese or five large scoops of ice cream. (Of course, this choice may *taste* the best, but there are obvious drawbacks to eating five scoops of ice cream every day!) In addition to its nutritional value as a developer of bones and organs, milk has been found to help people sleep. People who drink milk at night go to sleep more quickly, and sleep longer and sounder. This is because of the high content of the amino acid tryptophan, which makes serotonin, the neurotransmitter (brain chemical) associated with relaxation and calming.

Coffee contains several ingredients that may be harmful to the body. There are stimulants such as caffeine and the xanthines, as well as oils that seem to stimulate the secretion of excess acid in the stomach. And there are diuretics that eliminate water and some nutrients, such as calcium, from the body. Even two cups a day increases the risk of bone fractures[1]. A factor that may add to the risk of bone fractures is that people who drink more coffee usually drink little or no milk.

---

[1] E. Barrett-Connor, "Caffeine and bone fractures," *Journal of the American Medical Association*, January 26, 1994.

Caffeine is found in coffee, tea, and cola and many other soft drinks. Brewed coffee contains 100 to 150 milligrams of caffeine per cup (mg/cup), instant coffee about 90 mg/cup, tea between 45 and 75 mg/cup, and cola drinks from 40 to 60 mg/cup. Decaffeinated coffee is virtually free of caffeine, containing only two to four mg/cup. The therapeutic dose of caffeine given to people who have overdosed on barbiturates is 43 milligrams. Yet a cup of coffee contains up to 150 milligrams of caffeine!

Caffeine is a central nervous system stimulant. It elevates your blood pressure and constricts your blood vessels, both of which effects may assist in the development of high blood pressure. It has also been reported that excess caffeine in coffee, tea, and cola drinks can produce the same symptoms found in someone suffering from psychological anxiety, including nervousness, irritability, occasional muscle twitching, sensory disturbances, diarrhea, insomnia, irregular heartbeat, a drop in blood pressure, and occasionally failures of the blood circulation system.

Coffee is an irritant. The oils in coffee irritate the lining of the stomach and the upper intestines. People who drink two or more cups of coffee per day increase their chances of getting ulcers by 72 percent over non–coffee drinkers. Decaffeinated coffee is no more soothing to the ulcer patient than the regular blend, because both types increase the acid secretions in the stomach. Since an ulcer patient's acid secretion is not as high when caffeine alone is ingested (when compared to the acid levels after the ingestion of decaffeinated coffee), some other ingredient in coffee is thought to be responsible for these increased stomach acid levels.

Tea is not as irritating as coffee, but it does contain some caffeine and tannic acid, which can irritate the stomach. If you drink large amounts of tea, you should either take it with milk to neutralize the acid or add ice to dilute it. Green tea, the type commonly drunk in Asia, contains polyphenols, which appear to be antioxidants and may reduce cancer incidence. Black tea, the kind commonly drunk in Europe and America, has less of these protective substances[2]. Not much is known about the effects of herbal teas.

Alcohol contains seven calories per gram. These calories contain no nutritional elements, but they do contribute to your total caloric intake. Since alcoholic drinks are surprisingly high in calories, they contribute to the overweight problems of many individuals. People who drink alcoholic beverages and eat a balanced diet will probably consume too many calories. If they drink but cut down on eating, they may not develop a weight problem, but they will probably develop nutritional deficiencies that can result in severe illness. Alcohol is also a central nervous system depressant, which causes a decrease in one's metabolism.

---

[2] *University of California, Berkeley Wellness Letter*, January 1992, pp. 1–2.

In addition to the normal dangers of alcohol in creating alcoholism and destroying brain cells, there are other considerations in drinking. Beer or ale, because of their carbonation, have the effect of neutralizing stomach acid. This can increase the acids secreted by the stomach, causing ulcers.

Food Additives

Sugar is a negative for most people. In fact it is probably the most harmful additive to the foods that we in the United States eat. We average about 125 pounds of sugar per person per year. This gives us a lot of excess calories that, if not used for energy, will be stored as fat. As discussed previously, if we exceed our desired weight and become obese, we will have increased health risks.

Salt can be a dangerous food additive, yet most people do not consider adding salt to their food to be a health risk. But when you look at populations as a whole, it seems obvious that the higher the salt intake, the greater the frequency of high blood pressure.

Many manufacturers add salt to enhance the taste of food, and sodium is often high in processed or canned foods. While the desired intake is between one and two grams (1,000 and 2,000 milligrams), the average daily intake in America is five grams. The potential negative effect of a high sodium intake can be combated by ingesting a high level of potassium. However, the desired recommended daily allowance for potassium, 2.5 grams, is not met by the average American, who consumes only 0.8 to 1.5 grams daily. Most of our foods follow this same pattern—too high in sodium and too low in potassium.

Preservatives added to foods lengthen storage life and prevent disease-causing germs from multiplying. Most are harmless, and some give protection against intestinal cancers. Some, however, such as the nitrates in hot dogs, have been implicated in causing cancer. Nevertheless, the disease of botulism, which they prevent, is far more of a danger than that posed by the nitrates.

Vitamins and minerals have been added to food for years. In 1973, the Food and Drug Administration suggested that more iron be added to enrich flour after they found that iron is often low in our diets. Vitamins A and D are added to skim milk to make it nonfat milk—milk that has all of the nutrients of whole milk but without the fat. Vitamins A and D are fat soluble and stay in the fat when it is removed to make skim milk.

Vegetarianism

When vegetarians are careful about their dietary intakes, they may prove to be healthier than nonvegetarians. One study comparing healthy vegetarians to nonvegetarians found that healthy vegetarians had lower blood sugar and cholesterol levels than did their closely matched nonvegetarian counterparts.

Smart Shopping

Shopping for low-fat foods requires a sharp eye. If you are looking for a low-fat food, look at the total grams of fat, multiply by nine (nine calories per gram of fat), then divide that by the total number of calories in the food. (For example, if a food has three grams of fat, nine times that equals 27 total calories from fat. If the food has a total of 270 calories, then the percentage of fat calories is 10 percent.) If the food has one of the new food labels, it will list both the number of fat calories and the approximate percentage of fat calories per serving. You want to keep your daily total percentage of fat below 30 percent to decrease your risk of developing heart disease. Even better than the suggested maximum of 30 percent is keeping the total to 10 or 20 percent fat.

Many foods, particularly low-fat liquids such as salad dressings without oil, have replaced the oil with some gums. Guar, locust bean, and xanthine gums are soluble fibers that help remove cholesterol from the intestines. So you get a double advantage—no fat and some cholesterol-removal substances.

The food label lists ingredients according to their content in the product. The higher on the list of ingredients, the more of that item is present in the food. So if the product lists wheat flour first, there is no problem. But if it lists eggs or hydrogenated oils second, the food may be too high in fat. And if you are watching your sodium intake, remember to look for salt on the list.

Eating and Overeating

People eat to nourish their bodies. But in America many people eat to reduce stress. We may not be satisfied in our work, at school, or in our relationships, but we can be satiated with food. Filling our stomachs can make us feel that in at least one part of our lives we are totally satisfied. When we eat to relieve stress, we will probably take in more calories than we need for living—but even worse, stress eating often means junk foods. It is much more intelligent to play some volleyball to relieve stress.

Being overweight is a more common concern than is being underweight. While some people are overweight, some are obese. For example, 35 percent of women are 20 percent overweight[3]. Of people who are obese, one in 20 has a genetic factor or a problem in physical malfunctioning, such as an underactive thyroid, a problem with the hypothalamus, or one of the other centers of the brain that deals with whether or not we feel full or hungry. There are medical procedures that can help these people. In cases where the metabolism is slowed, such as by an underactive thyroid gland, doctors can administer the proper hormone to increase metabolism back into what is considered a normal range.

---

[3] *Harvard Women's Health Watch*, November 1994, p. 4.

Another cause of obesity is thought to be the number of fat cells in a person's body. This is known as the *set point theory*. It is thought that the more fat cells one has, the more one is driven to eat to maintain these fat cells. The number of fat cells one has is generally set after puberty.

For others, obesity is caused by overeating to an extreme degree. However, according to the Harvard University Nutrition Department, most people are overfat because they don't exercise, not because they overeat. Overeating coupled with a lack of exercise is a sure way to become obese.

Since it is the amount of body fat that a person carries that is the true culprit of disease, it is preferable to refer to this health risk as being overfat rather than being overweight. Many bodybuilders may be overweight when compared to the height/weight charts commonly used to measure health risks by insurance companies, but they are not overfat.

Determining if you are overfat can be done in several ways. The most common method is to look at yourself in a mirror. If you look fat, you may be fat. Another way is to pinch the fat you carry just below the skin. If you can pinch an inch, you are probably carrying too much fat. Professionals often use skin calipers to measure the amount of fat people carry in four to seven designated spots on the body, or they use underwater weighing or bioelectrical impedence.

Once your body fat percentage is determined, you can then find out what a healthy weight would be for you. Men are usually considered healthy if their body fat is in the range of 10 to 15 percent, while women are healthy if they fall between 18 to 25 percent body fat. Men are considered overfat if their body fat is over 20 percent, while women are overfat if their body fat is over 30 percent. Women require more fat than men do because of their menstrual cycle. If a woman falls below 12 percent body fat, she may become amenorrheic (lose her regular menstrual cycle).

Should You Lose Weight?

Before you decide to lose weight, you first need to determine whether your are overweight due to being overfat. From a health point of view, it is your proportion of fat and lean body mass that is most important.

How to Lose Weight

The wisest approach to losing weight would be to find out why you are overweight. If it is genetic, perhaps medical help is needed. If you eat because of stress, you should find another way to relieve stress, such as exercise or relaxation techniques or, if you must have something in your mouth, try gum or a low-calorie food. If your problem is a lack of exercise, start an effective exercise program. If you consume too many calories, you will need to change your diet.

Don't even start a weight-loss program if you are not willing to make lifestyle changes for the rest of your life. The great majority of dieters refuse to make such a commitment. That is why 40 percent of women and 25 percent of men are on a diet at any one time, and the average American goes on 2.3 diets a year, and it is also why 95 percent of dieters regain all of their lost weight within five years. The average diet is just not successful.

In all likelihood, if you adopt the habits of effective exercise and a low-fat and low-alcohol eating pattern, the pounds will drop off. Losing weight just for the sake of being thinner seldom works for very long. You have to determine whether you honestly want a healthier lifestyle or just to look better for the summer. A pattern of continually gaining and losing weight is frustrating and probably not worth the effort. But a true lifestyle change to healthy eating and regular exercise will pay many mental, physical, and social dividends.

We must recognize that the fat we wear comes primarily from the fat we eat. Because carbohydrates are so efficiently converted to sugar glucose, they are used first for energy in the body. To convert carbohydrates to fat, about 23 percent of the energy is used to make the conversion. Protein, if not used, will normally be converted into sugars and will be the second source of available energy. But the fat you eat uses only 3 percent of its food value in the conversion to body fat.

So 25 grams of carbohydrate, which will yield 100 calories (at 4 calories a gram), is reduced by 23 percent of the calories used to convert them to body fat. But fats consumed in your food are different. Eleven grams of fat (at nine calories per gram) is 99 calories, but it only takes 3 percent of those calories to convert it all to body fat, and 96 calories of body fat can be deposited. So 100 calories of carbohydrates, if not used for energy, will become about 8.5 grams of body fat, but 100 calories of fat from the diet will become about 10.75 grams of body fat.

To lose one pound of fat per week, you must have a net deficit of 500 calories per day; one pound of fat contains 3,500 calories. You may choose to achieve this solely by decreasing your food intake by 500 calories per day.

You could also choose to increase your activity level to burn off 500 calories a day. Keep in mind that it takes a great deal of energy to achieve this goal, and it can be dangerous for you to embark on such a strenuous exercise program if you are not currently exercising. It is best to combine calorie reduction with exercise to achieve your goal. Aerobic exercise will keep your metabolism up as you lose the fat, and you won't have to restrict your calories as much because you will be burning off energy each time you exercise.

Playing volleyball in a physical education class burns about .036 calories per pound per minute. For a 150-pound person, this is about 325 calories per hour. If you are playing hard volleyball such as in competitive games, this would be about .065 calories per pound per minute, or 585 calories per hour for a 150-pound person. An aggressive game of doubles in the sand would use even more calories.

We now know that calories are used both during and after exercise. The longer and more vigorous the exercise, the longer one's metabolism is increased, so that for more hours after the exercise is completed, the calorie expenditure will be increased over normal. While this increase in calories burned after one has finished exercising is not a large amount, it is still an increase over one's resting metabolism, and a calorie burned is a calorie burned!

Some people think that exercising will make them eat more. A quarter-mile to a mile of jogging or a good set of volleyball games will have no measurable effect on the total intake of calories. In fact, by exercising just before a meal, you can dull your appetite and decrease your desire for more calories.

Eating Disorders

Anorexia nervosa is starvation by choice. This is a disease primarily seen in young women. It afflicts nearly one in a hundred women, although 5 to 10 percent of its victims are male. In this disease, the person goes on a diet and refuses to stop, no matter how thin he or she gets. About one out of ten people who have this disorder end up starving themselves to death. The disease has a psychological basis, but its physical effects are very real. Medical care, usually hospitalization, is generally required.

After the anorexic begins the severe dieting routine, symptoms of starvation may set in, leading to a number of physical problems. Abnormal thyroid, adrenal, and growth hormone functions are not uncommon. The heart muscle becomes weakened. Amenorrhea occurs in women and girls due to the low percentage of body fat. Blood pressure may drop. Anemia is common due to the lack of protein and iron ingested. The peristalsis of the intestines may slow and the lining of the intestines may atrophy. The pancreas often becomes unable to secrete many of its enzymes. Body temperature may drop. The skin may become dry and there can be an increase of body hair in the body's attempt to keep itself warm. And for 10 percent of sufferers, the result is death.

Because dieting is such a common occurrence in our society, anorexia is often difficult to diagnose until the person has entered the advanced stages of the disease. However, other symptoms such as moodiness, being withdrawn, obsessing about food but never seen eating it, and constant food preparation may be observed by those close to the anorexic. Once diagnosed, there are a number of medical and psychological therapies that can be effective.

Bulimia, or *bulimia nervosa*, is more common than anorexia. The person with bulimia restricts calorie intake during the day, but binges on high-fat, high-calorie foods at least twice a week. Following the binge, the person purges in an attempt to get rid of the excess calories just consumed. Purging techniques include vomiting, laxatives, fasting, and excessive exercise. Some experts do not consider the behavior bulimic until it has persisted for about three months with two or more binges per week during that time. Estimates based on various surveys of college students and others indicate that between 5 and 20 percent of women may be bulimic. It is also more common among men than is anorexia.

Bulimia, like anorexia, stems from a psychological problem. However, in some cases there may also be a link to physical abnormalities. The neurotransmitters serotonin and norepinephrine seem to be involved, as does the hormone cholecystokinin, which is secreted by the hypothalamus and makes a person feel that enough food has been eaten.

Physical symptoms to look for depend on the type of purging technique used. The bulimic who induces vomiting can have scars on the back of the knuckles, mouth sores, gingivitis, tooth decay, a swollen esophagus, and chronic bad breath. The bulimic who uses laxatives has constant diarrhea, which can cause irreparable damage to the intestines. All bulimics run the risk of throwing off their electrolytes (minerals involved in muscle contractions) as a result of constant dehydration. It is this imbalance of electrolytes that can cause the bulimic to have abnormal heart rhythms and that can induce a heart attack.

Female athletes sometimes develop problems called the "female athletic triad,"[4] or a combination of eating disorders, osteoporosis, and amenorrhea. It is caused by the hard training practiced by competitive athletes or dancers and the desire to keep weight low, which often results in inadequate nutrition. Weight loss is sometimes achieved by bulimic methods. The result is weight that is too low, a loss of calcium from the bones, and a lack of healthy menstruation.

These problems are most likely to occur in activities in which low weight is an advantage, such as dancing, distance running, figure skating, and gymnastics, and it is more prevalent among athletes in individual sports than in team sports. Males, with the exception of competitive wrestlers, do not often experience the need to eat less. While this disorder doesn't generally affect volleyball players, you should be aware of the problem.

Fluid Replacement

Fluid replacement is essential if you sweat—and most serious volleyballers do. The ingredients of sweat change as you exercise. At the beginning, there are a number of salts excreted. Sodium chloride (common table salt) as well as potassium, calcium, chromium, zinc, and magnesium salts can be lost. As exercise continues, the amount of salts in the sweat is reduced because some of the body's hormones come into play. Aldosterone, for example, conserves sodium for the body. Consequently, the longer we exercise, the more our sweat resembles pure water.

A normal diet replaces all of the necessary elements lost in sweat. Drinking a single glass of orange or tomato juice replaces all or most of the calcium, potassium, and magnesium lost in exercise. In any case, most of us have plenty of sodium in our daily diets.

---

[4] Aurelia Nattiv, Barbara Drinkwater, et al. "The female athletic triad," *Clinics in Sports Medicine: The Athletic Woman*, W. B. Saunders: Philadelphia, 13(2), April 1994, pp. 405–418.

Fluid replacement drinks on the market are not usually the best choice. Water, the most needed element, is slowed in its absorption if the drink contains other elements such as salts and sugar. Water alone is therefore generally recommended for fluid replacement—and it is certainly less expensive. For those who want to replace water and sugars for energy, the best drinks are those that contain glucose polymers (maltodextrins). So if you are using fluid replacement drinks, check the label, then buy what you need—salts and/or sugars. Both caffeine (coffee, tea, and cola drinks) and alcohol dehydrate the body and should be avoided.

Self-Test

Write in the number that best describes your eating habits:

3—Almost always   2—Sometimes   1—Almost never

____ **1.** Do you eat three or more pieces of fruit per day? (Fruit juice counts as one piece.)

____ **2.** Do you eat a minimum of three servings of vegetables each day—including a green leafy or orange vegetable?

____ **3.** Do you eat three or four milk products (such as milk, cheese, yogurt) per day?

____ **4.** Do you eat a minimum of six servings of grain products (breads, cereal, pasta) each day?

____ **5.** Do you eat breakfast?

____ **6.** Do you eat fish at least three times per week?

____ **7.** Do you avoid fried foods, including potato chips and french fries?

____ **8.** Do you eat fast food fewer than three times per week?

____ **9.** Are the milk products you consume made from nonfat milk?

____**10.** Do you avoid high-sugar foods and highly refined carbohydrates such as sweet rolls, cookies, non-diet sodas, candy, etc.?

Your Score

25–30   You are balancing your diet well.

18–24   Your diet needs to be improved.

10–17   Your diet is unhealthy.

Bulimia Self-Test

Write "Never," "Sometimes," or "Often" to describe your weight-control practices:

____ 1. Is your life a series of constant diets?

____ 2. Do you vomit or take laxatives or diuretics to control your weight?

____ 3. Do you alternate periods of eating binges with fasts to control your weight?

____ 4. Does your weight fluctuate by as much as 10 pounds because of eating habits?

____ 5. Have you ever had a "food binge" during which you ate a large amount of food in a short period of time?

____ 6. If you "binged," was it on high-calorie food such as ice cream, cookies, donuts, or cake?

____ 7. Have you ever stopped a binge by vomiting, sleeping, or experiencing pain?

____ 8. Do you think your eating habits vary from the average person's?

____ 9. Are you out of control with your eating habits?

____10. Are you close to 100 pounds overweight because of your eating habits?

If you marked two or more of the above questions "Often," you may have a serious eating disorder called *bulimia*.

Where to Go for Help

Anorexia Bulimia Treatment Education Center: 800-33-ABTEC

Bulimia Anorexia Self-Help: 800-227-4785

Low-fat diet gourmet meals are possible. Send for the free *Metropolitan Cookbook*. Write to: Health and Welfare Department, Metropolitan Life Insurance Co., 1 Madison Avenue, New York, NY 10010) . Or buy the American Heart Association's cookbook.

Height and Weight Table: Men*

Height	Small Frame	Medium Frame	Large Frame
5'2"	128–134	131–141	138–150
5'3"	130–136	133–143	140–153
5'4"	132–138	135–145	142–156
5'5"	134–140	137–148	144–160
5'6"	136–142	139–151	146–164
5'7"	138–145	142–154	149–168
5'8"	140–148	145–157	152–172
5'9"	142–151	148–160	155–176
5'10"	144–154	151–163	158–180
5'11"	146–157	154–166	161–184
6'0"	149–160	157–170	164–188
6'1"	152–164	160–174	168–192
6'2"	155–168	164–178	172–197
6'3"	158–172	167–182	176–202
6'4"	162–176	171–187	181–207

*Weights at ages 25 to 59 based on lowest mortality. Weight in pounds according to frame (in indoor clothing weighing 5 lbs.; shoes with 1" heels).
Source: 1999 Metropolitan Life Insurance Company height and weight tables.

Height and Weight Table: Women†

Height	Small Frame	Medium Frame	Large Frame
4'10"	102–111	109–121	118–131
4'11"	103–113	111–123	120–134
5'0"	104–115	113–126	122–137
5'1"	106–118	115–129	125–140
5'2"	108–121	118–132	128–143
5'3"	111–124	121–135	131–147
5'4"	114–127	124–138	134–151
5'5"	117–130	127–141	137–155
5'6"	120–133	130–144	140–159
5'7"	123–136	133–147	143–163
5'8"	126–139	136–150	146–167
5'9"	129–142	139–153	149–170
5'10"	132–145	142–156	152–173
5'11"	135–148	145–159	155–176
6'0"	138–151	148–162	158–179

†Weights at ages 25 to 59 based on lowest mortality. Weight in pounds according to frame (in indoor clothing weighing 3 lbs.; shoes with 1" heels).
Source: 1999 Metropolitan Life Insurance Company height and weight tables.

Calories Burned with Various Activities

	Calories per pound per hour	Calories expended by 150 lb. person in 20 minutes
Sleeping	0.36	18.0
Sitting at rest	0.55	27.5
Sitting at work	0.60	30.0
Light exercise (housework)	1.00	50.0
Walking	1.20	60.0
Jogging	1.75	87.5
Volleyball (recreational six-person)	1.50	65.0
Volleyball (advanced doubles in sand)	4.14	207.0

Summary

1. Sensible eating requires some understanding of the science of nutrition.
2. Following the guidelines of the Food Pyramid will generally give a person an adequate diet.
3. Skim or nonfat milk is the best beverage.
4. Salt and sugar are the most common food additives.
5. Many people overeat and become overfat.
6. Most overfat people can lose weight through an effective diet and adequate exercise.
7. Eating disorders seem to be prevalent; anorexia nervosa and bulimia are the major eating disorders.

19

The Mental Side of Becoming a Better Player

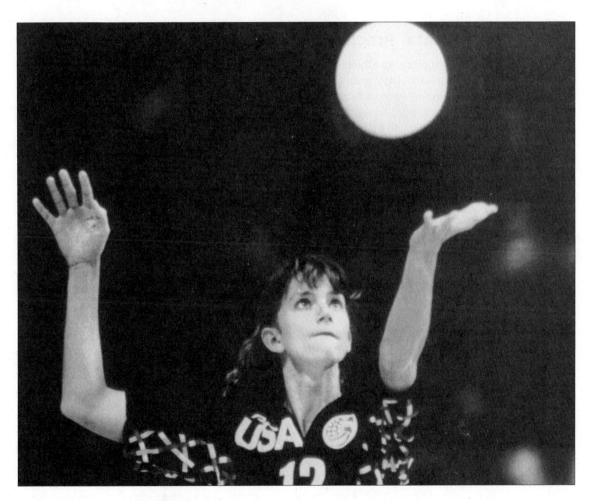

Outline

Wishing won't make you a better player. You must learn and practice the physical skills of volleyball. This practice will take place primarily on the court. While it is important to work out physically to condition your body, you can also become a better player at home by practicing mentally. There are many skills to learn in volleyball and there are so many ways to practice that you should always be able to help your game in some way.

Mental Practice

Championship athletes have known for years that mental practice can help performance. Only recently have sports psychologists refined methods of utilizing the mind's contribution to the game. *Mental imagery*, or *visualization*, are the names given to this type of mental practice. It can be done externally—observing volleyball players or a videotape, or imagining watching yourself from outside your body. (Golfer Jack Nicklaus calls this "going to the movies.") It can also be done internally—"feeling" yourself doing the action.

While mentally experiencing your game, you can practice your sets and spikes, your footwork, or even strategy and court positioning. You can practice whatever aspect of your game you would like to improve. If your service return is a problem, imagine yourself ready for it. The imaginary opponent tosses the ball and serves to your left. Feel yourself making the proper play. Move toward the ball, get your arms in proper position, watch the ball, and make the perfect pass. Think of keeping your head down and your eyes focused on the ball.

The following study serves to illustrate how mental imagery can help your game[1]. Basketball players were divided into two groups. The first group physically practiced 100 free throws per day, while the second group was placed in a dark, quiet room and told to imagine that they were successfully making 100 free throws. When the two groups were tested at the end of the study, the second group shot for a better percentage. Analysts believe that this resulted from the second group's mental imagery, in which they were successful in 100 percent of their shots, while the other group that was actually shooting missed some of their throws and therefore were not as confident when it came to the actual test.

When using this technique in volleyball, imagine yourself doing everything correctly from start to finish, being sure to include a successful outcome. Perform the action at full speed in your mind, and use as many senses as you can. For example, if you are going to play before a large crowd, you might play crowd noise on a tape player in the background as you mentally practice your skills.

---

[1] Daniel Elon Smith, *Evaluation of an Imagery Training Program with Intercollegiate Basketball Players*, unpublished doctoral dissertation, University of Illinois at Urbana–Champaign, 1986, pp. 91–104.

Checklist for Mental Imagery

1. Watch top-level volleyball players or videotapes of volleyball skills.
2. Be the star in your own movie by closing your eyes and performing skills to perfection in your mind.
3. Always see yourself completing all aspects of the skill perfectly, including a successful finish.
4. Practice all aspects of the game mentally as well as physically.
5. Always be positive in your instructions to yourself.

Relaxation

Relaxation is another essential facet of good volleyball. Practice taking a slow, deep breath before preparing to serve. This can help clear your mind so you can concentrate on the serve, and can also help to relax your muscles between periods of action. Relaxed muscles are more prepared for the quick movements essential to playing the game of volleyball. Tense muscles tend to inhibit smooth, efficient activities and speed up the onset of fatigue.

To teach yourself to get the most out of relaxation and deep breathing, sit quietly in a chair with your eyes closed and concentrate on slowly taking and releasing deep breaths. You can say to yourself "breathe in, breathe out," or repeat a nonsense syllable such as "om" or "one." Concentrating on this syllable repetition is designed to help you relax by eliminating all tension-causing thoughts from your mind. By "not thinking" as you concentrate on your breathing, your muscles will relax and your blood pressure can be lowered. If other

 Checklist for Learning to Relax

1. Sit completely relaxed in a comfortable chair in a quiet room.
2. Close your eyes.
3. Slowly take in and release a deep breath while repeating a meaningless syllable.
4. The meaningless syllable repetition should help you to relax by blocking all tension-causing thoughts from your mind.
5. Don't worry if other thoughts come into your mind—just get back into your breathing pattern and your repetition of nonsense syllables.

thoughts come into your mind, return to your breathing pattern and verbal repetition. This is similar to the practice of meditation, and is the basis for many of the benefits to be gained from that practice.

After you have learned to relax while sitting calmly in a quiet place, the next step is to transfer that ability to volleyball practice, both on and off the court. You should be relaxed whenever you practice mental imagery, and you should also be able to relax on the court. A relaxed body is more ready to react than a tense body.

Since deep breathing and "not thinking" are important to total relaxation, you can breath deeply when you are tense during a match. Breathing deeply before serving or between rallies will help you to relax. If there is time and you have perfected the relaxation response, you can take a few seconds to close your eyes, repeat a meaningless syllable, and breathe deeply. This will give you a quick mental and physical rest.

Concentration

Concentration is the third major area of mental practice. You must have a specific focus in order to play at your maximum potential. That point of focus will vary during a rally.

Generally the most important area on the court to concentrate on is the ball. Failure to focus on the ball all the way to the point of contact and while it is on your hand or arm is probably the most common and critical error at every level of volleyball. Slow-motion studies reveal that most people take their eyes off of the ball when it is still four to six feet away from them. They look at where they want to hit the ball instead of concentrating on the point of contact of the ball and the body.

As you have noted earlier in the text, it is sometimes necessary to switch your focus of concentration, such as when blocking—from pass, to setter, to spiker. You must know where to focus in each situation—on the ball or on a segment of a player.

When concentrating on something, always keep it positive, such as "Watch the ball" or "I am relaxed." Negative thinking is counterproductive and can

 Checklist for Concentration

1. Know what or who should be your focus of concentration.
2. If your focus is the ball, focus on it from the first possible moment until after the ball has left your body.
3. If your focus is to change, such as from pass, to setter's arm action, to spiker, know the sequence and practice shifting your focus.

cause stress. The player who is thinking "I better not miss another serve" is setting him- or herself up for missing the next serve.

Goal Setting

Another important aspect of the mental side of the sport is *setting both long-term and short-term goals.* Short-term goals assist in achieving long-term goals.

After you decide on your long-term goals, make plans to achieve them. An example of a long-term goal is a desire to be the champion of your club or class tournament, or perhaps making the Olympic team.

Short-term goals are more measurable. They usually involve improving the specific skill that will enable you to achieve your long-term goal. Examples of short-term goals are improving your floater serve to the back corner or learning to time your jump for the spike.

Once you've set a goal, develop a practice schedule designed to increase your chances of attaining that goal. For example, if you want to increase in your ability to spike the ball, then, in addition to on-the-court repetition of the shot, you can also include mental practice. Visualize different sets—some low, some high, some making you move from your desired position.

With visual practice, you can start your physical practice. Have a partner set you some balls. Analyze what you have done right and wrong on your practice spikes. Then replace the negative with the positive in your mental practice.

Summary

1. The complete volleyball player must make use of his or her maximum mental potential. There are various ways to improve one's volleyball off the court.
2. Mental preparation includes:
   - *Imagery.* A person visualizes the techniques and the game situations that may be encountered.
   - *Relaxation.* It helps a player avoid tension and perform at a higher level.
   - *Concentration.* The player focuses on the ball all the way to the point of contact.
3. Goal setting is important for all areas of our lives. Effectively done when planning for improvement in volleyball, it can speed up one's improvement in skills and in enjoyment of the game.

Appendix **A**

ABRIDGED INTERNATIONAL VOLLEYBALL RULES

FACILITIES AND EQUIPMENT

PLAYING AREA: The playing area includes the playing court and the free zone. It shall be rectangular and symmetrical.

1.1 DIMENSIONS

The playing court is a rectangle measuring 18 x 9 m, surrounded by a free zone which is a minimum of 3 m wide on all sides. The free playing space is the space above the playing area which is free from any obstructions. The free playing space shall measure a minimum of 7 m in height from the playing surface. For FIVB World Competitions, the free zone shall measure a minimum of 5 m from the sidelines and 8 m from the end-lines. The free playing space shall measure a minimum of 12.5 m in height from the playing surface. For the senior World Championships and Olympic Games, the free zone shall measure a minimum of 6 m from the sidelines and 9 m from the end-lines.

1.2 PLAYING SURFACE

1.2.1 The surface must be flat, horizontal, and uniform. It must not present any danger of injury to the players. It is forbidden to play on rough or slippery surfaces.

1.3 LINES ON THE COURT

All lines are 5 cm wide. They must be of a light and different color from the floor and from any other lines.

1.3.2 Boundary lines

Two sidelines and two end-lines mark the playing court. Both side and end-lines are drawn inside the dimensions of the playing court.

1.4   ZONES AND AREAS

Front Zone

On each court the front zone is limited by the axis of the center-line and the attack-line drawn 3 m back from that axis (its width included). For FIVB World Competitions, the attack-line is extended by the addition of dotted lines from the sidelines, with five 15 cm short lines 5 cm wide, drawn 20 cm from each other to a total length of 1.75 m. The front zone is considered to extend beyond the sidelines to the end of the free zone.

Service Zone

The service zone is a 9 m wide area behind the end-line (the end-line excluded). It is laterally limited by two short lines, each 15 cm long, drawn 20 cm behind the end-line as an extension of the sidelines. Both short lines are included in the width of the service zone. In depth, the service zone extends to the end of the free zone.

Substitution Zone

The substitution zone is limited by the extension of both attack-lines up to the scorer's table.

2.1   HEIGHT OF THE NET

2.1.1 Placed vertically over the center-line there is a net whose top is set at the height of 2.43 m for men and 2.24 m for women.

2.1.2 Its height is measured from the center of the playing court. The net height (over the two sidelines) must be exactly the same and must not exceed the official height by more than 2 cm.

2.6   ADDITIONAL EQUIPMENT

All additional equipment is determined by FIVB regulations.

3.   BALLS

3.1   STANDARDS

The ball shall be spherical, made of a flexible leather case with a bladder inside made of rubber or a similar material.

- Its color should be uniform and light.
- Its circumference is 65-67 cm and its weight is 260-280 g.
- Its inside pressure shall be 0.30 to 0.325 kg/cm2 (294.3 to 318.82 mbar or hPa.

3.2   UNIFORMITY OF BALLS

3.3 All balls used in a match must have the same standards regarding circumference, weight, pressure, type, etc.

4.3   EQUIPMENT

A player's equipment consists of a jersey, shorts, socks, and sport shoes.

4.3.1. Jerseys, shorts, and socks must be uniform, clean, and of the same color for the team.

4.3.2 The shoes must be light and pliable with rubber or leather soles without heels.

4.3.3 Players' jerseys must be numbered from 1 through 18. The number must be placed on the jersey at the center of the front and of the back.

The color and brightness of the numbers must contrast with the color and brightness of the jerseys.

5.   **TEAM LEADERS**

Both the team captain and the coach are responsible for the conduct and discipline of their team members.

5.1   **CAPTAIN**

Prior to the match, the team captain signs the scoresheet and represents his/her team in the toss.

5.1.2 During the match, the team captain acts as the game captain while in play. When the team captain is not playing on the court, the coach or the captain him/herself must assign another player on the court to assume the role of game captain. This game captain maintains his/her responsibilities until either he/she is substituted, the team captain returns to play, or the set ends. When the ball is out of play, only the game captain, of all the team members, is authorized to speak to the referees . . . to ask for an explanation of the application or interpretation of the Rules, and also to submit the requests or questions of his/her team-mates. If the explanation does not satisfy the game captain, he/she must immediately indicate to the referee his/her disagreement. Hereby he/she reserves the right to record an official protest on the scoresheet at the end of the match

PLAYING FORMAT

6.   **TO SCORE A POINT, TO WIN A SET AND THE MATCH**

6.1   **TO SCORE A POINT**

6.1.1 Playing fault: Whenever the team makes a playing action contrary to these Rules, or otherwise violates them, a playing fault is whistled by one of the referees. The referees judge the faults and determine the penalties according to these Rules:

   a)   If two or more faults are committed successively, only the first one is counted.

   b)   If two or more faults are committed by opponents simultaneously, a double fault is called and the rally is replayed.

6.1.2 Consequences of a fault: The consequence of a fault is loss of rally; the opponent of the team committing the fault wins the rally with one of the following consequences:

   a)   If the opponent served, it scores a point and continues to serve.

   b)   If the opponent received the service, it gains the right to serve, without scoring a point (side-out), except in the deciding set.

   c)   In the deciding set (the 5th), when the receiving team wins the rally, it gains the right to serve, but also scores a point (Rally-Point Scoring).

6.2   TO WIN A SET

6.2.1 A set is won by the team which first scores 15 points with a minimum lead of two points. In the case of a 14-14 tie, play is continued until a two-point lead is achieved (16-14, 17-15).

6.2.2 In the first four sets there is a point limit at 17: that is, after a 16-16 tie the team scoring the 17th point wins the set with only a one-point lead.

6.2.3 In the deciding set (the 5th) there is no point limit: in the case of a 14-14 tie, play is continued until a two-point lead is reached.

6.3   TO WIN THE MATCH

6.3.1 The match is won by the team that wins three sets.

6.3.2 In the case of a 2-2 tie, the deciding set (the 5th) is played with Rally-Point Scoring (Rule 6.1.2.c).

6.4   DEFAULT AND INCOMPLETE TEAM

6.4.1 If a team refuses to play after being summoned to do so, it is declared in default and forfeits the match with the result 0-3 for the match and 0-15 for each set.

6.4.2 A team that, without justifiable reason, does not appear on the playing court on time is declared in default with the same result as in Rule 6.4.1.

6.4.3 A team that is declared incomplete for the set or for the match (Rule 7.3.1.a), loses the set or the match. The opposing team is given the points, or the points and the sets needed to win the set or the match. The incomplete team keeps its points and sets.

7.   STRUCTURE OF PLAY

7.1   THE TOSS

Before the match the first referee carries out a toss to decide upon the first service and the sides of the court in the first set. If a deciding set is to be played, a new toss will be carried out.

7.1.1 The toss is taken in the presence of the two team captains.

7.1.2 The winner of the toss chooses either:
a)   The right to serve or to receive the service, or
b)   The side of the court.
The loser takes the remaining choice.

7.1.3 In the case of consecutive warm-ups, the team that has the first service takes the first turn at the net.

7.2   WARM-UP SESSION

7.2.1 Prior to the match, if the teams have previously had a playing court at their disposal, each team will have a 3-minute warm-up period at the net; if not, they may have 5 minutes each

7.2.2 If both captains agree to warm up at the net together, the teams may do so for 6 or 10 minutes, according to Rule 7.2.1.

7.3   TEAM LINE-UP

7.3.1 a)   There must always be six players per team in play.
b)   The team's starting line-up indicates the rotational order of the players on the court. This order must be maintained throughout the set.

7.4   POSITIONS

At the moment the ball is hit by the server, each team must be positioned within its own court in the rotational order (except the server).

7.4.1 The positions of the players are numbered as follows:

The three players along the net are front-row players and occupy positions 4 (front-left), 3 (front-center), and 2 (front-right). The other three are back-row players occupying positions 5 (back-left), 6 (back-center) and 1 (back-right).

7.4.2 a)   Each back-row player must be positioned further back from the net than the corresponding front-row player.

b)   The front-row players and the back-row players, respectively, must be positioned laterally in the order indicated in Rule 7.4.1.

7.4.3 The positions of players are determined and controlled according to the positions of their feet contacting the ground as follows:

a)   Each front-row player must have at least a part of his/her foot closer to the center-line than the feet of the corresponding back-row player.

b)   Each right (left) side player must have at least a part of his/her foot closer to the right (left) sideline than the feet of the center player of his row.

7.5   POSITIONAL FAULT

7.5.1 The team commits a positional fault, if any player is not in his/her correct position at the moment the ball is hit by the server (Rules 7.3 and 7.4).

7.5.2 If the server commits a serving fault at the execution of the service (Rules 13.4 and 13.7.1), the server's fault prevails over a positional fault.

7.5.3 If the service becomes faulty after the service hit, (Rule 13.7.2), it is the positional fault that will be counted.

7.5.4 A positional fault leads to the following consequences:

a)   The team is sanctioned with loss of rally (Rule 6.1.2).

b)   Players' positions are rectified.

7.6   ROTATION

7.6.1 Rotational order is determined by the team's starting line-up and controlled with the service order and players' positions throughout the set. Substitution requires the referee's authorization (for limitations of substitution, see Rule 8.1).

7.6.2 When the receiving team has gained the right to serve, its players rotate one position clock-wise: the player in position 2 rotates to position 1 to serve, the player in position 1 rotates to position 6, etc.

7.7   ROTATIONAL FAULT

7.7.1 A rotational fault is committed when the service is not made according to the rotational order (Rule 7.6.1). It leads to the following consequences:

a)   The team is sanctioned with a loss of rally (Rule 6.1.2).

b)   Players' rotational order is rectified.

7.7.2 Additionally, the scorer should determine the exact moment when the fault was committed, and all points scored subsequently by the team at fault shall be canceled. The opponent's points remain valid. If that moment cannot be determined, no point(s) cancellation takes place, and loss of rally is the only sanction.

8.   SUBSTITUTION OF PLAYERS

A substitution is the act by which a player leaves the court and another player occupies his/her position.

8.1   LIMITATIONS OF SUBSTITUTIONS

8.1.1 Six substitutions is the maximum permitted per team per set. One or more players may be substituted at the same time.

8.1.2 A player of the starting line-up may leave the game and re-enter, but only once in a set, and only to his/her previous position in the line-up.

8.1.3 A substitute player may enter the game, but only once per set in the place of a starting line-up player, and he/she can only be replaced by the player whom he/she replaced.

8.3   SUBSTITUTION FOR EXPULSION

An expelled or disqualified player (Rules 21.2.3 and 21.2.4) must be replaced through a legal substitution. If this is not possible, the team is declared incomplete (Rule 6.4.3).

8.4   ILLEGAL SUBSTITUTION

8.4.1 A substitution is illegal if it exceeds the limitations indicated in Rule 8.1.

8.4.2 When a team has made an illegal substitution and the play has been resumed (Rule 9.1), the following procedure shall apply:

a)   The team is penalized with loss of rally.

PLAYING ACTIONS

9.   STATES OF PLAY

9.1   BALL IN PLAY

The ball is in play from the moment of the hit of the service authorized by the first referee.

9.2   BALL OUT OF PLAY

The ball is out of play at the moment of the fault which is whistled by one of the referees; in the absence of a fault, at the moment of the whistle.

9.3   BALL "IN"

The ball is "in" when it touches the floor of the playing court including the boundary lines (Rule 1.3.2).

9.4   BALL "OUT"

The ball is "out" when:

a)   The part of the ball which contacts the floor is completely outside the boundary lines.

b)   It touches an object outside the court, the ceiling, or a person out of play.

c) It touches the antennae, ropes, posts or the net itself outside the side-bands.

d) It crosses the vertical plane of the net totally or even partly outside the crossing space:
- during service, or
- into the opponent's court.

10. PLAYING THE BALL

Each team must play within its own playing area and space (except Rule 11.1.2). The ball may, however, be retrieved from beyond the free zone.

10.1 TEAM HITS

The team is entitled to a maximum of three hits (in addition to blocking, Rule 15.4.1), for returning the ball. If more are used, the team commits the fault of "four hits." The hits of the team include not only intentional hits by the players, but also unintentional contacts with the ball.

10.1.1 Consecutive contacts: A player may not hit the ball two times consecutively (except Rules 10.2.3, 15.2.1 and 15.4.2).

10.1.2 Simultaneous contacts: Two or three players may touch the ball at the same moment under the following circumstances:

a) When two (three) teammates touch the ball simultaneously, it is counted as two (three) hits (with the exception of blocking). If they reach for the ball, but only one of them touches it, one hit is counted. A collision of players does not constitute a fault.

b) When two opponents touch the ball simultaneously over the net and the ball remains in play, the team receiving the ball is entitled to another three hits. If such a ball goes "out", it is the fault of the team on the opposite side.

c) If simultaneous contacts by two opponents lead to a "catch" (Rule 10.2.2), it is a "double fault" (Rule 6.1.1.b) and the rally is replayed.

10 1.3 Assisted hit: Within the playing area, a player is not permitted to take support from a teammate or any structure/object in order to reach the ball. However, a player who is about to commit a fault (touch the net or cross the center-line, etc.) may be stopped or held back by a teammate.

10.2 CHARACTERISTICS OF THE HIT

10.2.1 The ball may touch any part of the body.

10.2.2 The ball must be hit, not caught and/or thrown. It can rebound in any direction.

10.2.3 The ball may touch various parts of the body, provided that the contacts take place simultaneously.

Exceptions:

a) At blocking, consecutive contacts (Rule 15.2.1) may be made by one or more blocker(s) provided that the contacts occur during one action.

b) At the first hit of the team (Rules 10.1 and 15.4.1), the ball may contact various part of the body consecutively provided that the contacts occur during one action.

10.3.   FAULTS IN PLAYING THE BALL
   a)   Four hits: A team hits the ball four times before returning it (Rule10.1).
   b)   Assisted hit: A player takes support from a teammate or any structure/object within the playing area in order to reach the ball (Rule 10.1.3).
   c)   Catch: A player does not hit the ball, and the ball is caught and/or thrown (Rule 10.2.2).
   d)   Double contact: a player hits the ball twice in succession or the ball contacts various parts of his/her body in succession (Rule 10.2.3).

11.   BALL AT THE NET
11.1   BALL CROSSING THE NET
11.1.1 The ball sent to the opponent's court must go over the net within the crossing space. The crossing space is the part of the vertical plane of the net limited as follows:
   a)   Below, by the top of the net
   b)   At the sides, by the antennae and their imaginary extension
   c)   Above, by the ceiling
11.1.2 The ball that has crossed the net plane to the opponent's free-zone (Rule 12) totally or partly outside of the crossing space may be played back within the team hits provided that:
   ■   The opponent's court is not touched by the player
   ■   The ball when played back crosses the net plane again outside the crossing space on the same side of the court.
   The opponent team may not prevent such action.
11.1.3 The ball is "out" when it crosses completely the lower space under the net.
11.2   BALL TOUCHING THE NET
   While crossing the net (Rule 11.1.1), the ball may touch it except at the service.
11.3   BALL IN THE NET
11.3.1 A ball driven into the net may be recovered within the limits of the three team hits (Rule 10.1), except the service.
11.3.2 If the ball rips the mesh of the net or tears it down, the rally is canceled and replayed (Exception: the service, Rule 11.2).
12.   PLAYER AT THE NET
12.1   REACHING BEYOND THE NET
12.1.1 In blocking, a blocker may touch the ball beyond the net, provided that he/she does not interfere with the opponents' play before or during the latter's attack-hit (Rule 15.3).
12.1.2 A player is permitted to pass his/her hand beyond the net after an attack-hit, provided that the contact has been made within his/her own playing space.
12.2   PENETRATION UNDER THE NET
12.2.1 It is permitted to penetrate into the opponents' space under the net, provided that this does not interfere with the opponents' play.

12.2.2 Regarding penetration into the opponent's court, beyond the center-line:

   a)   To touch the opponent's court with a foot(feet) or hand(s) is permitted, provided that some part of the penetrating foot(feet) or hand(s) remains either in contact with or directly above the center-line.

   b)   To contact the opponent's court with any other part of the body is forbidden.

12.2.3 A player may enter the opponent's court after the ball goes out of play (Rule 9.2).

12.2.4 A player may penetrate into the opponent's free zone provided that he/she does not interfere with the opponents' play.

12.3   CONTACT WITH THE NET

12.3.1 Contact with the net is a fault, except when a player not attempting to play the ball accidentally touches the net.

12.3.2 Once the player has hit the ball, he/she may touch the post, rope or any other object outside the total length of the net provided that it does not interfere with play.

12.3.3 When the ball is driven into the net and causes it to touch an opponent, no fault is committed.

12.4   PLAYER'S FAULTS AT THE NET

A fault at the net occurs when:

   a)   A player touches the ball or an opponent in the opponents' space before or during the opponents attack-hit (Rule 12.1.1).

   b)   A player penetrates into the opponents' space under the net interfering with the latter's play (Rule 12.2.1).

   c)   A player penetrates into the opponents' court (Rule 12.2.2.b).

   d)   A player touches the net (Rule 12.3.1).

13.   SERVICE

The service is the act of putting the ball into play by the back-right player, placed in the service zone (Rule 13.4.1).

13.1   FIRST SERVICE IN A SET

13.1.1 The first service of the first set, as well as that of the deciding set (the 5th) is executed by the team determined by the toss (Rule 7.1).

13.1.2 The other sets will be started with the service of the team that did not serve first in the previous set.

13.2   SERVICE ORDER

13.2.1 The players must follow the service order recorded on the line-up sheet (Rule 7.3.1).

13.2.2 After the first service in a set, the player to serve is determined as follows:

   a)   When the serving team wins the rally, the player (or his/her substitute) who served before, serves again.

   b)   When the receiving team wins the rally, it gains the right to serve and rotates before actually serving (Rule 7.6.2). The player who moves from the front-right position to the back-right position will serve.

13.3   AUTHORIZATION OF THE SERVICE

The first referee authorizes the service after having checked that the two teams are ready to play and that the server is in possession of the ball.

13.4   EXECUTION OF THE SERVICE

13.4.1 The ball shall be hit with one hand or any part of the arm after being tossed or released from the hand(s), and before it touches any other part of his/her body or the playing surface.

13.4.2 At the moment of the service hit or take-off for a jump service, the server must not touch the court (the end line included) or the ground outside the service zone. After the hit, he/she may step or land outside the service zone, or inside the court.

13.4.3 The server must hit the ball within 5 seconds after the first referee whistles for service.

13.4.4 A service executed before the referee's whistle is canceled and repeated.

13.5   SERVICE ATTEMPT

13.5.1 If, after the ball has been tossed or released, the server lets it fall on the ground without touching it, it is considered to be a service attempt.

13.5.2 After a service attempt, the referee authorizes the service again, without any delay, and the server must execute it within the next 3 seconds.

13.5.3 One and only one service attempt is permitted for each service.

13.6   SCREENING

13.6.1 The players of the serving team must not prevent their opponent, through screening, from seeing the server or the path of the ball.

13.6.2 Individual screen: A player of the serving team makes an individual screen if he/she waves his/her arms, jumps or moves sideways, etc., when the service is being executed, and the ball is served over him/her.

13.6.3 Collective screen: A team makes a collective screen when the server is hidden behind a group of two or more team-mates, and the ball is served over them.

13.7   SERVING FAULTS

13.7.1 Serving faults: The following faults lead to a change of service, even if the opponent is out of position (Rule 13.8.1). The server:

a)   Violates the service order (Rule 13.2)

b)   Does not execute the service properly (Rule 13.4)

c)   Violates the rule of service attempt (Rule 13.5)

13.7.2 Serving faults after hitting the ball: After the ball has been correctly hit, the service becomes a fault (unless a player is out of position) if the ball (Rule 13.8.2):

a)   Touches a player of the serving team or fails to cross the vertical plane of the net

b)   Touches the net (Rule 11.2)

c)   Goes "out" (Rule 9.4)

d)   Passes over an individual or collective screen (Rule 13.6)

13.8   SERVING FAULTS AND POSITIONING

13.8.1 If the server makes a serving fault (improper executions, wrong rotational order, etc.) and the opponent is out of position, it is the serving fault which is penalized.

13.8.2 Instead, if the execution of the service has been correct, but the service subsequently becomes faulty (touches the net, goes out, screened, etc.), the positional fault has taken place first and is penalized.

14.   ATTACK-HIT

14.1.1 All actions which direct the ball towards the opponents, with the exception of service and block, are considered as attack-hits.

14.1.2 During an attack-hit, tipping is permitted if the contact is clean and the ball is not accompanied by the hand.

14.1.3 An attack-hit is completed the moment the ball completely crosses the vertical plane of the net or is touched by an opponent.

14.2   RESTRICTIONS OF THE ATTACK-HIT

14.2.1 A front-row player may complete an attack-hit at any height, provided that the contact with the ball has been made within the player's own playing space (except Rule 14.2.4).

14.2.2 A back-row player may complete an attack-hit at any height from behind the front zone:

    a) At his/her take-off, the player's foot(feet) must neither have touched nor crossed over the attack-line.

    b) After his/her hit, the player may land within the front zone (Rule 1.4.1).

14.2.3 A back-row player may also complete an attack-hit from the front zone, if at the moment of the contact any part of the ball is below the top of the net.

14.2.4 No player is permitted to complete an attack-hit on the opponents' service, when the ball is in the front zone and entirely higher than the top of the net.

14.3   ATTACK-HIT FAULTS

Attack-hit faults occur when:

    a) A player hits the ball within the playing space of the opposing team (Rule 14.2.1).

    b) A back-row player completes an attack-hit from the front zone, if at the moment of the hit the ball is entirely above the top of the net (Rule 14.2.3).

    c) A player completes an attack-hit on the opponent's service, when the ball is in the front zone and entirely above the top of the net (Rule 14.2.4).

15.   BLOCK

15.1   BLOCKING

15.1.1 Blocking is the action of players close to the net to intercept the ball coming from the opponents by reaching higher than the top of the net.

15.1.2 Block attempt: A block attempt is the action of blocking without touching the ball.

15.1.3 Completed block: A block is completed whenever the ball is touched by a blocker. Only front-row players are permitted to complete a block.

15.1.4 Collective block: A collective block is executed by two or three players close to each other and is completed when one of them touches the ball.

15.2   BLOCK CONTACT

15.2.1 Consecutive (quick and continuous) contacts may occur by one or more blockers, provided that the contacts are made during one action.

15.2.2 These contacts may occur with any part of the body.

15.3   BLOCKING WITHIN THE OPPONENT'S SPACE

In blocking, the player may place his/her hands and arms beyond the net provided that this action does not interfere with the opponents' play. Thus, it is not permitted to touch the ball beyond the net until an opponent has executed an attack-hit.

15.4   BLOCK AND TEAM HITS

15.4.1 A block contact is not counted as a team hit (Rule 10.1). Consequently, after a block contact, a team is entitled to three hits to return the ball.

15.4.2 The first hit after the block may be executed by any player, including the one who has touched the ball during the block.

15.5   BLOCKING THE SERVICE

To block an opponent's service is forbidden.

15.6   BLOCKING FAULTS

A blocking fault occurs when:

a)   The blocker touches the ball in the opponents' space either before or simultaneously with the opponents' attack-hit (Rule 15.3).

b)   A back-row player completes a block or participates in a completed block (Rules 15.1.3 and 15.1.4).

c)   Blocking the opponents' service (Rule 15.5).

d)   The ball is sent "out" off the block (Rule 9.4).

e)   Blocking the ball in the opponent's space from outside the antenna.

INTERRUPTIONS AND DELAYS

16.   REGULAR GAME INTERRUPTIONS

Regular game interruptions are time-outs and player substitutions.

16.1   NUMBER OF REGULAR INTERRUPTIONS

Each team is entitled to a maximum of two time-outs and six player substitutions per set.

16.2   REQUEST FOR REGULAR INTERRUPTIONS

16.2.1 Interruptions may be requested by the coach or the game captain, and only by them. The request is made by showing the corresponding hand signal when the ball is out of play and before the whistle for service.

16.2.2 A request for substitution before the start of a set is permitted, and should be recorded as a regular substitution in that set.

16.3   SEQUENCE OF INTERRUPTIONS

16.3.1 The request for one or two time-outs, and one request for player substitution by either team may follow one another, with no need to resume the game.

16.3.2 However, a team is not authorized to make consecutive requests for player substitution during the same interruption of play. Two or more players may be substituted during the same interruption (Rule 8.11).

16.4   TIME-OUTS and TECHNICAL TIME-OUTS

16.4.1 A time-out lasts for 30 seconds.

16.5   PLAYER SUBSTITUTION

(For limitations, see Rule 8.1.)

16.6   IMPROPER REQUESTS

16.6.1 It is improper to request an interruption:

a)   During a rally or at the moment of, or after the whistle to serve by a non-authorized team member

b)   For player substitution before the game has been resumed from a previous substitution by the same team

c)   After having exhausted the authorized number of time-outs and player substitutions

16.6.2 Any improper request that does not affect or delay the game shall be rejected without any sanction unless repeated in the same set.

17.   GAME DELAYS

17.1   TYPES OF DELAYS

An improper action of a team that defers resumption of the game is a delay and includes, among others:

a)   Delaying a substitution

b)   Prolonging other interruptions, after having been instructed to resume the game

c)   Requesting an illegal

d)   Repeating an improper request in the same set

e)   Delaying the game by a player in play

17.2   SANCTIONS FOR DELAYS

17.2.1 The sanction of "delay warning" or "delay penalty" is a team sanction.

17.2.2 The first delay by a team in a set is sanctioned with a "delay warning."

17.2.3 The second and subsequent delays of any type by any player or other member of the same team in the same set constitute a fault and are sanctioned with a "delay penalty": loss of rally.

18.   EXCEPTIONAL GAME INTERRUPTIONS

18.1   INJURY

18.1.1 Should a serious accident occur while the ball is in play, the referee must stop the game immediately and permit medical assistance to enter the court. The rally is then replayed.

18.1.2 If an injured player cannot be substituted, legally or exceptionally the player is given a 3-minute recovery time, but not more than once for the same player in the match. If the player does not recover, his/her team is declared incomplete (7.3.1.a).

18.2   EXTERNAL INTERFERENCE

If there is any external interference during the game, play has to be stopped and the rally is replayed.

18.3   PROLONGED INTERRUPTIONS

18.3.1 If unforeseen circumstances interrupt the match, the first referee, the organizer and the Control Committee, if there is one, shall decide the measures to be taken to re-establish normal conditions.

19.   INTERVALS AND CHANGE OF COURTS

19.1   INTERVALS

All intervals between sets, including the one between the 4th and 5th sets, last three minutes. During this period of time, the change of courts and line-up registrations of the teams on the scoresheet are made.

19.2   CHANGE OF COURTS

19.2.1 After each set, the teams change courts, with the exception of the deciding set. Other team members change benches.

19.2.2 In the deciding set, once a team reaches 8 points, the teams change courts without delay and the player positions remain the same. if the change is not made at the proper time, it will take place as soon as the error is noticed. The score at the time that the change is made remains the same.

PARTICIPANTS' CONDUCT

20.   REQUIREMENTS OF CONDUCT

20.1   SPORTSMANLIKE CONDUCT

20.1.1 Participants must know the "Official Volleyball Rules" and abide by them.

20.1.2 Participants must accept referees' decisions with sportsmanlike conduct, without disputing them. In case of doubt, clarification may be requested only through the game captain.

20.1.3 Participants must refrain from actions or attitudes aimed at influencing the decisions of the referees or covering up faults committed by their team.

20.2   FAIR-PLAY

20.2.1 Participants must behave respectfully and courteously in the spirit of fair-play, not only towards the referees, but also towards other officials, the opponents, teammates and spectators.

20.2.2 Communication between team members during the match is permitted.

21.   MISCONDUCT AND ITS SANCTIONS

21.1   MISCONDUCT

Incorrect conduct by a team member towards officials, opponents, teammates or spectators is classified in four categories according to the severity of the offense.

21.1.1 Unsportsmanlike conduct: argumentation, intimidation, etc.

21.1.2 Rude conduct acting contrary to good manners or moral principles, expressing contempt.

21.1.3 Offensive conduct: defamatory or insulting words or gestures.

21.1.4 Aggression: physical attack or intended aggression.

21.2   SANCTION SCALE

Depending on the severity of the offense, according to the judgment of the first referee, the sanctions to be applied are:

21.2.1 Misconduct warning: For unsportsmanlike conduct, no penalty is given but:

    a)   The team member concerned is warned against repetition in the same match.

    b)   The warning is recorded on the scoresheet.

    c)   Repeated unsportsmanlike conduct is sanctioned with loss of rally.

21.2.2 Misconduct penalty

    a)   For rude conduct, the team is penalized with the loss of rally.

    b)   The penalty is recorded on the scoresheet.

21.2.3 Expulsion

    a)   Repeated rude conduct in the same match is sanctioned by expulsion.

    b)   The team member who is sanctioned with expulsion must leave the Competition Control Area for the rest of the set.

    c)   The second expulsion of the same team member is regarded as a disqualification.

    d)   The penalty is recorded on the scoresheet.

21.2.4 Disqualification

    a)   Offensive conduct or aggression is sanctioned by disqualification.

    b)   The team member who is sanctioned with disqualification must leave the Competition Control Area for the rest of the match.

    c)   The penalty is recorded on the scoresheet.

21.3   APPLICATION OF SANCTIONS

21.3.1 The repetition of misconduct by the same team member in the same set or match is sanctioned progressively as shown in the sanction scale (Rule 21.2)

21.3.2 Disqualification due to offensive conduct or aggression does not require a previous sanction.

21.4   MISCONDUCT BEFORE AND BETWEEN SETS

Any misconduct occurring before or between sets is sanctioned according to Rule 21.2 and sanctions apply in the following set.

Appendix B

Volleyball Resource Directory

VIDEOS

Contact:
Marv Dunphy
Pepperdine University
Malibu, CA 90265
213-456-4517

BOOKS

USVBA Official Guide (Annual)
(All rules and pertinent data related to the game.)
3595 E. Fountain
Colorado Springs, CO 80910
719-578-4750

USVBA Equipment Manual
c/o Chairman of Equipment
3208 Newcastle Drive
Dallas, TX 75220
214-357-3655

For the most current lists of books and videos, contact:

Volleyball One Sales Company
15392 Assembly Lane, Suite C
Huntington Beach, CA 92649
714-898-4432

Quality Coaching
Box 11051
Burbank, CA 91510
800-541-5489, 818-842-6800

MAGAZINES AND PERIODICALS

Volleyball USA
Official publication of U.S. Volleyball Association, published quarterly
Subscription:
4 issues per year, $10.00 U.S. subscribers
4 issues per year, $20.00 international
VIP
1227 Lake Plaza Dr., Suite B
Colorado Springs, CO 80906
800-275-8782

Coaching Volleyball
Publication of AVCA
Subscription: U.S.
VIP
1227 Lake Plaza Dr., Suite B
Colorado Springs, CO 80906
800-275-8782

Beach Volleyball Magazine
2049 Century Park East, Suite 5086
Los Angeles, CA 90067

Volleyball
Box 566
Mt. Morris, IL 61054
815-734-6309

Volleyball Monthly
Box 3137
San Luis Obispo, CA 93403

Midwest Volleyball Magazine
3052 N. Laramie
Chicago, IL 60641
312-779-0319

ORGANIZATIONS

United States Volleyball Association
3595 E. Fountain
Colorado Springs, CO 80910
Phone: 719-637-8300   Fax: 719-635-0426

Association of Volleyball Professionals
2049 Century Park East, Suite 5086
Los Angeles, CA 90067

American Volleyball Coaches Association
122 Second Avenue, Suite 217
San Mateo, CA 94401

Federation of Outdoor Volleyball Associations
Box 5246
Carson, CA 90749

INTERNET SITES

General Index of Topics:
http://www.volleyball.org/general/index.html

U.S.A. Volleyball:
http://www.volleyball.org/usav/index.html

Olympic Volleyball:
http://www.volleyball.org/olympics/index.html

International Volleyball (Federation International of Volleyball):
http://www.volleyball.org/fivb/index.html

Professional Volleyball:
http://www.volleyball.org/pros/index.html

College Volleyball:
http://www.volleyball.org/college/index.html

Other Sites:
http://www.volleyball.org/www_sites/index.html

Index